A HAPPY AND HEALTHY PREGNANCY

THE FIRST-TIME MOM'S GUIDE TO TAKING CONTROL OF HER HEALTH AND OVERCOMING COMMON PREGNANCY CHALLENGES

AMANDA JAMES

TABLE OF CONTENTS

My friend was so excited when she received a positive pregnancy test. She and her husband had been eager to start their own family for years, but they kept putting it off until they found "the right time."

As you already know, there is no right time! If you keep waiting for everything to be perfect, you might never feel ready to have a baby. But my friend was convinced that if she got pregnant when everything else in her life was just so, the pregnancy would also go off without a hitch.

She spent several months preparing for maternity leave, decorating the nursery, and reading every parenting book she could get her hands on. She was so happy, flitting around like a busy bee.

But when she was seven months pregnant, her enthusiasm waned. She used to give me all sorts of updates about doctor's visits, paint colors, nursery themes, and more. When it stopped, I was so nervous for her. I was sure she had gotten some bad news and didn't know how to share it.

Since I have an extensive background studying families, parenting, and pregnancy, I wanted to let her know I was there for her no matter what was going on. I took her out to lunch and very diplomatically broached the subject of her pregnancy. I braced myself to hear bad news so I wouldn't get emotional and make things even harder for her.

"I'm going to have a baby," she said, looking at me with genuine fear in her eyes.

I was so confused! Of course, she was having a baby! She'd just spent seven months excitedly centering her life around that fact! I gently questioned her more so I could understand what she was feeling.

"Like, I'm actually going to have a baby. I'm going to have to give birth! I'm going to have to raise it! I don't know how to do this!"

I reassured her that she had already started preparing for the baby. After all, she had been reading so many parenting books!

"I don't believe those books," she told me. "They're either too fluffy, telling me I'll love the baby no matter what and just naturally know what to do. Or they're too matter-of-fact and recommend calling the doctor and doing extensive research on every little thing. Not only is the advice from one book directly contradicting another book, but neither of those approaches feels right to me."

I can't tell you how excited I was to use my extensive pregnancy and parenting knowledge to help my friend overcome her predicament. We worked together to take stock of all she had already done, what aspects of pregnancy she felt confused by, and why she felt that way.

When I visited my friend and her new baby, I couldn't believe how peaceful they both looked. As new mothers do, my friend kept beaming, but she was directing these amazing smiles at me!

"I couldn't have done it without you," she told me. "There's so much information out there that I totally overloaded myself! You stripped it down to the facts and gave me the information I could use, and I can never thank you enough."

I assured her that I did it because I loved her and cared for her well-being, but also that she could repay me by letting me hold her sweet baby!

I couldn't get my friend's words and smiles out of my head. I was so happy that I had helped her, but I kept thinking about the conflicting information she had read. It's possible to go out there and get the facts—plenty of pregnancy books cover medical concerns, and your OB-GYN is skilled enough to help you with any questions and problems you may have.

And it's also possible to find plenty of books that proclaim you'll be a natural mother as soon as the baby is born. When you hold your baby, you'll know exactly what to do with them. While it's nice when that instant love connection happens between you and your baby, it's not always the case.

I started thinking about all of the information I shared with my friend and thought I should compile it to help other women. Not only is your body is experiencing changes, but your mind and emotions also experience ups and downs during pregnancy.

Having that explained matter-of-factly might help pregnant women because they won't have to figure out if they're struggling or if what they're going through is normal.

I also had so much advice about what to eat to help both your body and your mind. What if I combined all my tips for physical, emotional, and mental care during pregnancy into one book? Like a one-stop-shop for pregnant women! Perhaps distilling this knowledge into one book would be more helpful than expecting a woman to tackle an extensive reading list, especially on top of everything she's already going through while pregnant!

So welcome to my one-stop-shop, the book that will help you have a happy and healthy pregnancy, from the minute you get a positive result to giving birth—and beyond! (Ever heard of the fourth trimester? It's real, and I can help you handle it!)

I'm so excited to share my knowledge with you to empower you on your pregnancy journey. I've spent years studying family sociology, including family units, marriage, parenting, and, of course, pregnancy. I understand the changes your body, mind, and emotions will go through on this journey. I can help you keep them under control while still balancing your relationship with your partner, extended family, and friends.

The most important thing to remember is that this is the most magical time of your life—you're about to become a mother! Your life will change in so many unique ways, so stay positive, take a deep breath, and get ready to learn. Remember, I'm here for you, holding your hand and helping you get everything under control.

"WHAT IS HAPPENING TO ME?" — MUST-HAVE KNOWLEDGE ABOUT THE CHANGES THAT OCCUR DURING PREGNANCY

As soon as you knew you wanted to become a mother, you had some ideas of what would happen. It seems like pregnancy in the media is commonly portrayed in two main ways. It can be a heavenly experience where you walk around with that special glow, happily rubbing your belly and talking to your baby. Or it can take a significant toll on you physically, mentally, and emotionally. You're walking around with a rat's nest of hair on your head, throwing up every morning, and dealing with constant aches and pains.

The reality is that you'll most likely have a mix of those two experiences. Some days can be pretty hard; then, you'll catch a break and be so excited about how your life is changing. You might have a rough first trimester, then breeze through the rest of your pregnancy. It's a different experience for everyone, and I think that's why so many of the other books on the market have trouble genuinely speaking to women. They're trying to give general information that can apply to everyone, but really, you should know the nitty-gritty of everything, so you know what to expect.

Whether you have a peaceful pregnancy or tough times, your entire being is going to undergo some pretty significant changes, so let's explore each of them more in-depth.

PHYSICAL CHANGES

I don't want to rain on your parade, but there is no way to put it gently: there is a laundry list of things that will change with your body physically. Most women know and accept that their belly will expand, their ankles will swell, and eventually, they'll have to get the baby out of their body, which brings about its own changes. But there's more to it than that.

Some changes happen to protect your growing baby, like differences in hormone levels, weight gain, and energy.

Hormones

Hormones influence more bodily functions than you realize. Human chorionic gonadotropin (HCG) is a hormone that the placenta produces to prepare your body to accept the egg's implantation. It's most potent during the first trimester and is predominantly responsible for nausea you'll most likely experience during that time.

Human placental lactogen (hPL) is another hormone produced by the placenta. It stimulates the growth of your milk glands, which will prepare you to breast-feed your baby. As your breasts start to grow during pregnancy, you might be uncomfortable with the size and pressure you feel.

Pro tip: buy nursing bras early in the pregnancy and start wearing them. You don't have to be breast-feeding to benefit from the comfort they provide. They can also be more affordable than buying new bras in larger sizes because you can wear them as your breasts grow during pregnancy as well as when you're nursing. If you invest in larger bras, they won't be conducive to easy breastfeeding, so you'll end up buying nursing bras anyway.

On that note, buying maternity clothes early in your pregnancy can be helpful because you can pick up items as you find good deals. And you can wear them whenever you want! Maternity clothes are comfortable, so as your body changes, you'll appreciate how soft and forgiving maternity clothes are. Many women I know have started wearing them in their second or third month and continued wearing them long after giving birth!

But let's get back to the hormones that are causing all of this discomfort. Your body will produce more estrogen when you're pregnant to help keep you and your baby healthy. Over time, you'll also produce more progesterone, which will loosen your joints so your body can make room for your uterus as it expands, and also so you'll be more comfortable when giving birth.

Some of these hormones, such as progesterone, can be balanced with supplements. We'll explore that aspect of your health more in chapter four when we get to diet.

Weight

Every woman knows to expect weight gain with pregnancy; after all, you're growing a human in your belly! But the weight won't necessarily be restricted to your stomach, so that can be hard to adjust to. Women can gain anywhere from 25 to 35 pounds during pregnancy, and nowhere near all of that is your baby!

Weight gain usually happens during your second and third trimester, as you're getting hungrier and needing more calories to support both you and your growing baby. Though seeing your body change so drastically can be challenging, it's important to remember that your body is doing what your baby needs, so there's no need to diet while you're pregnant. You can make healthy food choices and exercise in approved ways to help keep your weight gain under control. We'll address both of those issues in future chapters.

Most of the weight you gain in your third trimester is water retention. It will make your ankles, hands, and feet swell, which can feel tight and uncomfortable. There's no solution to this problem, so you're better off trying to kick back and relax a little. Even though the issue is water retention, don't get confused and think that means your body has enough or too much water—you still need to stay hydrated!

Circulation

Since you're growing another person, your body will produce more blood during pregnancy to support you both. You can help increase the volume of your blood by eating iron-rich foods. I'll share a list of my favorites in the chapter about diet.

This increase in blood volume means your veins will be larger to accommodate the volume. You'll be susceptible to varicose veins and hemorrhoids. While varicose veins can look bad and feel itchy or uncomfortable, they're harmless in terms of your overall health.

Hemorrhoids are more painful and can be distressing since you might find blood in your stool as a result, and no one wants to see blood in the toilet during pregnancy! To prevent them, you can eat plenty of fiber and drink a lot of water to keep your stool soft. Moving around and being active more than you sit can also help prevent this pain. If you're suffering from hemorrhoids, talk to your doctor about treatments or supplements that can help.

Having more blood in your body will also make your kidneys and urinary system work harder to keep the blood clean and rid it of waste. You'll also experience frequent urination due to the increase of blood, along with pressure on your bladder. Even with frequent urination, you're more susceptible to urinary tract infections and yeast infections during pregnancy.

These changes in circulation can affect your blood pressure and make you feel dizzy. To combat the dizziness, make sure you're eating enough to keep your blood sugar stable, drink plenty of water, and always be careful when you're getting up from a lying or sitting position.

Taste, Smell, and Digestion

Digestion also changes when you're pregnant, as you might experience during morning sickness. Nausea is incredibly common, but so are extreme cravings and food aversions. It's common during your first trimester to have a metallic taste in your mouth as your body gets used to the constant changes. When this taste goes away, you might find yourself craving foods you never really enjoyed before. Or you might no longer love your favorite meals!

Your body is fine-tuning its senses to prevent you from eating anything that might make you sick or harm your baby, so it's best to just go with the flow as your tastes change. The recommended foods in chapter four will appeal to the more general taste buds and give you all the nutrients you need.

Your sense of smell can change as well. You might be able to smell something from far away, and you'll be more likely to have extreme reactions to these smells. Even if you previously weren't offended by certain scents, your elevated pregnancy hormones might make it so that certain smells make you feel sick or cause headaches.

Even if you've never had trouble with indigestion and heartburn, you can experience this during pregnancy. It's common during the third trimester when the baby has grown and is pushing on your stomach. While the foods you eat may be causing indigestion, you can also try to prevent that sensation by eating smaller meals more often. Doing this keeps your stomach from getting too full, so the baby can't push on it as much. If your heartburn is excruciating, ask your doctor about antacids that are safe to take during pregnancy.

Hair, Skin, and Nails

Pregnancy hormones might take you for a ride, but your hair, skin, and nails can benefit from this uptick in hormones. Your hair might get fuller during pregnancy, so appreciate it while you can! Some women experience hair loss in the fourth trimester as their hormones level out. You won't go bald or anything; it's just your body's way of balancing your hormones and getting back to normal growth, but it's good to know ahead of time that your hair can take you on such a roller coaster!

Along with your hair getting fuller and more robust, your nails will also grow faster than usual. Due to hormones, it's kind of hit or miss whether your nails will be stronger or more likely to break easily. Still, just like your hair, this is a temporary condition that will even out after you give birth.

During the first part of pregnancy, you might find that your skin has the "pregnancy glow" we've all heard so much about. This "glow" happens as your body experiences a rush of hormones. While it's usually a positive side effect, it, unfortunately, goes away as your body begins to level out your hormones and assign them to the necessary tasks.

Over time, you might develop dark patches of skin on your face. This is called melasma and will most likely go away after you give birth. You can use prescription creams on the dark patches with your doctor's approval, but the easiest way to treat them is by limiting your exposure to the sun and wait it out.

Your nipples will also get darker during pregnancy, and as your breasts grow, you might see more veins through the skin than you usually do. You might also notice the hair between your navel and pubic region darken. This is called linea nigra and will fade after you give birth, as your hormones balance.

Since your body is expanding, your skin might feel itchy as it stretches. You can use lotion to ease this sensation. After you take a bath or shower, gently pat yourself dry with a towel instead of rubbing. Apply lotion to your itchy areas (or your whole body) while you're still a little damp to really lock in the moisture. Your skin will thank you!

Speaking of skin, stretch marks are likely to appear as your stomach, breasts, hips, buttocks, and thighs grow. As your skin stretches, these marks might be red or pink, but they usually fade to light pink or white over time. Using lotion on your skin can also help prevent stretch marks.

Various Pains

After reading about all of these physical changes, it will come as no surprise to learn that your body will be experiencing various pains throughout this time. Your body has a lot of adjusting to do to accommodate your little one! While these pains can be uncomfortable and frustrating, know that most of them are natural because your body is expanding and changing for the best.

Backaches are incredibly common in pregnancy. You're carrying more weight in your stomach than usual, so your back muscles are having to compensate. Gentle massages can help ease these pains. You can also wear a maternity support band that helps distribute your weight evenly, so your back won't strain. Being active can also help; just make sure you're doing approved exercises for each trimester. You'll learn more about these in chapter three.

As the baby grows, it might put pressure on your sciatic nerve, sending shooting pains through your hips and legs. The pain is temporary and usually goes away on its own after the baby is born. Massages can help ease the discomfort during pregnancy, but if the problem persists past the fourth trimester, consult your doctor for help.

You might feel many other pains throughout your pregnancy, but keep in mind that they are temporary as your body balances itself. These discomforts might include:

- leg cramps
- nosebleeds and bleeding gums
- numb or tingling sensations in your extremities
- blurry vision
- overheating
- dehydration
- exhaustion

Hopefully, you found this section informative rather than scary and intimidating. Much of the advice in later chapters will help keep you healthy and active so that many of these concerns might not affect you. It's better to know what's possible than be blindsided because not only will you be mentally prepared for these pains you also won't let them impact your already fragile emotional state.

EMOTIONAL CHANGES

Thinking about becoming pregnant can be emotional enough; you're imagining a little one who embodies the best of you and your partner, picturing how they fit into your life, and daydreaming about what they might become as they grow up. The physical changes should not overshadow emotions you experience during pregnancy because your emotional health is just as important as your physical health!

Hormonal changes will impact your emotions just as they do your body, but also, the scope of change you're going through is enough to affect you emotionally! Your entire life is changing. You're bringing a new life into the world. You're going to grow this life in your body, give birth to it, and raise it. All of that is major, and all of it will make you emotional. It's a lot of adjustment, even if you feel completely prepared for parenthood.

The human chorionic gonadotropin (HCG) produced by your placenta to help the egg implant does more than impact you internally; it can also affect your emotions by making you feel incredibly peaceful or moody. Yes, it's absolutely that broad in its influence! It can also make you feel exhausted, and that fatigue can cause brain fog. It can be frustrating when you have trouble focusing on work or a simple task, but your body is trying to manage so many changes that it only makes sense that your mind is distracted as well. This fog is usually prevalent during the first trimester, like morning sickness, and eases throughout the pregnancy.

Estrogen makes you feel happy and gives you a peaceful sense of well-being. A mixture of other hormones fluctuating with estrogen can make you feel moody, easily irritable, and ready to cry at the drop of a hat. It's strange not feeling in control of your emotions and not knowing why you feel sad all of a sudden, but all you can do is ride the wave. It helps to eat healthily and be active because you'll increase your endorphins and serotonin, but that won't magically cure you of mood swings. The best way to cope is to make sure your partner is aware of these changes and won't feel attacked as you experience them. An understanding partner will make the whole process easier on you because if they take your mood swings personally, you'll be at risk for many pointless arguments!

However, your partner might love some of these emotional changes. During the second trimester, the increased blood flow can make your sexual organs feel more sensitive, so they'll appreciate your friskiness. Since your belly is still smaller during this time, but your breasts are growing, you'll most likely feel incredibly sexy—and your partner will see this in you as well. This is definitely one of the changes you'll want to enjoy while you can!

Another positive emotional change during pregnancy that often comes during the third trimester is a nesting instinct. As you near childbirth, you begin the exciting process of preparing a comfortable and loving environment for your baby. Scientists aren't sure if this is a real hormonal change taking place in your body, but studies have shown that your brain's reward system activates as you approach giving birth.

Your physical body has put in so much effort to provide a healthy space for your baby that it's now ready to create a comfortable space in your home. The third trimester is also when you're having baby showers, which opens a whole new set of emotions as you see the people who love and care about you come together to help you prepare for your baby.

You're getting gifts, baby-proofing the house, putting together a crib and rocking chair, and making space for your baby in your life. Many women also find that they enjoy cooking and cleaning more during this period. You've had six months to prepare for your baby internally, but now that your body is coasting towards giving birth, you want to get a grip on controlling some external factors of your home life as well.

Mood swings aren't always temporary. Pregnancy can cause depression in women who have a prior history of it, but depression can also appear in women who have previously felt well-balanced. Because mood swings are such a common character-istic of pregnancy, many women write off their depression as caused by pregnancy, but it can be more severe than that. Consult your doctor or a mental health professional if you feel like your emotions are more unstable than usual. Though eating well and exercising can help you balance your emotions, there's nothing wrong with asking for help, especially if you think your well-being is at stake.

It's also easy to fall into a pit of despair based on body image issues. Your body is changing so much in ways you might not have expected when you considered pregnancy. It can be easy to feel frustrated with your body and feel like it's failing you.

While the last section gave you some ways to combat physical pain, the best solution regarding your emotional reaction to pain and changes is to stay positive. It might not sound like much, but reframing your pain can help you accept it. Instead of feeling like your body is ugly and failing you, view it as making the necessary, natural changes needed to stay healthy while giving birth to a new life. You might still experience some physical discomfort, but you'll understand the greater purpose of the pain.

Not all emotional changes are due to hormones and your changing body. You're aware of how much your life will change after giving birth, so it's normal to worry about the future. Any problems you have with your partner or other family members might be exacerbated when you're pregnant. Having a baby can cause you to question strained relationships and boundaries with others. While your relationship with a family member might be troublesome, and you feel equipped to handle that, approaching it as a new parent with a baby to protect might have you second-guessing all you know.

Since pregnancy and giving birth are significant uncertainties for first-time moms, anxiety is a common emotion to experience for nine months. Anxiety can be a somewhat positive emotion because it gets your adrenaline going and helps you be more aware of possible problems around you. However, if your anxiety is constantly more negative than positive, it can spiral into fear instead of motivating you.

Fear is a common emotion pregnant women experience. You're worried about miscarriages, and the act of giving birth, and how healthy you and your baby will be throughout the process. You're scared of all of the problems that could affect the baby after birth and how prepared (or not) you feel to care for the baby.

A support system is crucial to getting through these problems. Talk to your partner about how you'll establish boundaries with family members and friends when it comes to your baby. While everyone will want to meet your little one, it's more than okay to set time limits on visits or restrict people who seem physically or emotionally unwell.

Not every woman will experience the same emotional changes, but it's essential to be aware of the possibilities. If you experience any negative emotion for more than two weeks, discuss it with your doctor so you can both be mindful of the situation. You might feel like you're asking too much of your partner by pulling them into your emotions as well, but having a solid support system can make a huge difference in how you experience your pregnancy. It's better to talk about your emotions with your partner than to keep them inside and feel resentful about everything you're going through.

So many pregnant women are focused on the well-being of their baby and growing family that they let their self-care slack, but you need to be healthy to care for your baby, whether you're still pregnant or have already given birth. It's known how negatively postpartum depression can affect women, but it's often overlooked that prenatal depression is also detrimental to women's health. We'll explore postpartum depression more in the chapter about the fourth trimester, so you'll be aware of how emotions balance after giving birth.

These emotional changes you'll experience will fluctuate throughout your pregnancy, just like your hormonal changes. Sometimes it can be a relief to know you'll be pregnant for nine months because you'll have time to think of many potential issues and work to find solutions to them, but don't be surprised if you don't have all of the answers. You might think your relationship with your mother-in-law will smooth out once you have her grandchild, but she might be as toxic as ever in ways you couldn't imagine.

Becoming a parent doesn't mean you'll have all of the answers, so take all of your emotional changes in stride and know that you have your entire life to learn. If you ever feel like your emotions are too much to manage during pregnancy or after giving birth, talking to your doctor or a mental health professional can help you understand what's going on. It's better to ask for help than to suffer silently.

MENTAL CHANGES

Some of the previously mentioned emotional problems can blur the line with mental issues, so it's essential to be aware of both aspects of your body during pregnancy. Feeling extreme emotions can affect your mental state and compound into severe problems of depression, anxiety, and stress, which, in turn, will impact your physical well-being.

Mental health involves how you process information throughout your daily life, while emotional health refers to how you react to this information. There is a way to balance your mental health while still having strong emotions, especially during pregnancy. While you can use the terms interchangeably, there are differences that can help you better understand what is happening.

Health professionals separate the two by saying that mental health is the brain's hardware, while emotional health is the software. That means you can use and treat your mental health without needing to change your emotional health.

But your overall mental state might change due to your pregnancy. Most women are very excited to be pregnant, but even then, negative thoughts can slip in. Some women are too anxious to feel excited about their pregnancy because they're worried about what could go wrong, and that's okay, too, in moderation.

Society expects all women to be excited about their pregnancy, to the extent that women who don't feel excited or don't immediately bond with their baby after birth feel shamed. This can send an emotionally fragile pregnant woman into a spiral, so I'm here to tell you that there is no "normal" mental state for pregnancy. If you feel happy the entire nine months, up and down for nine months, or worried for nine months, that's normal for you. All that matters is that you're caring for your body and your baby.

When you're thinking about how your life will change after having a baby, it's understandable that you may worry. There are so many unknowns in prenatal care, giving birth, and taking your baby home. You might have medical worries. You might doubt your ability to be a parent. If you had anxiety before your pregnancy, you might find your fluctuating hormones exacerbate it.

Your body produces more estrogen and progesterone to make a more inviting environment for your baby, so while it's comforting that your body is doing what it needs to do, it can be uncomfortable when you have to deal with the side effects. These hormones, in particular, affect your brain's neurotransmitters, which in turn ramp up your emotions.

Neurotransmitters are the chemicals in your brain that communicate with your body so it will complete necessary functions without you having to manually do it, like keeping your lungs breathing and keeping your heart beating.

Specific neurotransmitters, like serotonin, influence your emotions. Serotonin is a positive hormone that promotes a general feeling of well-being or calmness. Still, when your other hormones fluctuate, your body might not produce enough serotonin to balance you out.

While you can't control how your hormones affect you, you can try to be as positive as possible. That doesn't mean you should ignore anything that feels "off" with your physical or emotional state, but there's no need to worry about every little thing.

Remember that your body knows what to do, so as long as you're taking care of yourself, your baby will be fine. Listen to your doctor and follow their recommendations for food and exercise and try to let some of the other worries go. This guide will help prepare you for things that can happen during pregnancy, but it will also empower you to push through the uncertainties and recognize your capabilities.

2

THE STRENGTH OF A MOTHER — EMPOWERING YOURSELF TOWARD AN AMAZING PREGNANCY

When you're preparing for motherhood, you might feel like you need to have total control over your life and, by association, your baby's life. Becoming a mother is a significant sacrifice, so of course, you're going to want to ensure you're doing all you can to make the best life for your baby.

However, with all of the uncertainties in pregnancy, maintaining control can be tough to manage and easily stress you out if you try to do so. To be in control, you want to manage your pregnancy, which is possible if you're eating right and exercising. You can also control the supplies you're getting to prepare for your baby's arrival and how you're saving money to secure your financial future.

But you can't control everything that happens to you, so it's essential to have some flexibility. You can be in control and still roll with the punches. How you react to changes or issues in your pregnancy can impact how in control you still feel when you face them.

ACCENTUATING THE POSITIVE

When you worry about everything during pregnancy, from the food you're eating to the vitamins you're taking to the colors you're choosing for the nursery's walls, that stress takes a physical, emotional, and mental toll on you. It can negatively impact your sleep cycle, your emotional well-being, and how you eat.

Instead of worrying about those matters, flip them into positives. Ensure you're eating the right foods to nourish your body and acknowledge that vitamins mean you're ensuring your baby will get what they need. Instead of being self-conscious about your body changing, know that it is making the necessary changes to carry your baby.

When you reframe your worries as positive situations, you're boosting your mental and emotional health. In turn, this benefits your physical health because you'll sleep better and feel more inclined to eat healthy foods when you're not worrying about the uncontrollable.

It's crucial to balance your positivity just as you do everything in moderation in pregnancy. Toxic positivity can be more stressful than worrying because you're so fixated on believing that everything is perfect. If you don't allow yourself to feel worries or bad feelings, you'll miss out on the full pregnancy experience. Reframing worries as positives doesn't mean you're scolding yourself for having the concerns in the first place, and it doesn't mean you're wrong to think them. It means you're reframing them as something positive before you let the stress of that worry drive you to anxiety.

No matter where you are in your pregnancy journey, you can benefit from changing your mindset. If you haven't been eating healthy meals for a month or more into your pregnancy, you don't have to double down and accept that as the reality for the remainder. You can reframe it as saying, "It's never too late to change my habits for the better." Every day is a new start where you can change yourself and improve your future.

You might also worry about what kind of parent you'll be. It sounds like a cliché, but it's true: if you're worried about being a good parent, you're going to be a good parent. The act of worrying shows you care. Even if you don't have positive parent role models from your childhood, you can still be a good parent to your offspring. You can educate yourself by reading books about pregnancy and parenting. (You're already doing a great job with that!) You can also find parents or experts you admire and analyze what parenting qualities they have that you would like to adopt.

If you're having trouble framing your worries as positives, don't force the issue. You can distract yourself from the concerns entirely by doing something good for yourself, like eating a healthy snack, doing an energizing exercise, or going for a walk. Making these good choices will boost your serotonin and adrenaline, so your worries might melt away naturally! And if not, you can always feel better that you're taking positive actions toward your health instead of letting the worries consume you.

Remember, over 90% of pregnancies that go beyond the first trimester result in healthy childbirth (Kelly, 2018). Even for the 10% at risk of complications, medical intervention has come such a long way that your doctor and nurses can easily handle problems. Worrying over something that isn't likely to happen will only stress you out at a time when you need to be relaxing and taking care of yourself.

Being positive doesn't mean you have to let go of all control and fully embrace an "ignorance is bliss" mindset, but it does help if you can let go of your expectations and go with the flow. Many women have a particular birth experience in mind, and they worry about what will happen if it doesn't go according to plan. Instead of worrying, accept that whatever birth happens and results in holding your child in your arms is going to be great, even if it's not *your* plan. Letting go of some of that control and focusing on the outcome can help you feel more relaxed through your entire pregnancy. It doesn't mean you have to stop planning anything. Just make sure you're open to the possibilities.

PARTNER SUPPORT

Making all of these life changes, including accentuating the positive, will be even more manageable if you have your partner's support. It's easy to feel like you're all alone in what you're experiencing, despite having a partner. After all, no one else is feeling what you feel while you carry and grow your baby. But letting people in on what you're experiencing, worried about, and looking forward to can help you feel more upbeat throughout your entire pregnancy.

If you're feeling stressed, you need to make sure your partner knows. Together you can find the root of your anxiety and work with each other to eliminate it. Ideally, your partner will be picking up the slack to make things easier for you. Of course, certain things will fall on you since you're the pregnant one, but you should never feel like the weight of the world is on your shoulders.

When your partner can help decrease your stress, you'll be happier. Your physical health will also improve, and your baby will feel these results in the best way possible. So, your partner helping manage all the difficulties they can is better for everyone!

Partners can support you by accompanying you to doctor's visits. Sometimes this isn't possible due to work schedules, but if at all possible, this is a massive benefit for pregnant women that you should take advantage of. Even if you feel completely prepared for a doctor's visit with a list of questions and concerns, it's nice to have someone there to hold your hand and be a second set of ears. Remember all of those hormones crashing through your body? They make pregnancy brain real, so even if you're taking extensive notes in your appointments, you're likely to forget something after you leave and not be able to find it in your notes or your memory. If your partner is with you, you know they heard the same information and can help you remember.

It's also helpful to have your partner attend doctor's visits because you might have to make choices about prenatal tests. While you can always ask for time to research an examination and talk it over with your partner, it's nice to have them there as the doctor explains it so you can both make an informed decision. And when the doctor performs the test, you'll want your partner by your side for moral support!

After your appointments, go for lunch, dinner, or even just to a cafe to spend time together. Taking time to be together can strengthen your relationship and help you feel more supported.

Childbirth classes are also a great way to spend time together and prepare for the baby. In these classes, you'll learn how to breathe during labor, prepare your body to give birth, and more. You'll have a chance to meet other couples going through the same thing as you, which can help expand your support system. These classes allow your partner to more fully understand everything you're going through and will have to do during labor. These classes also ensure your partner will know how to be a source of support when you're giving birth.

Very often, childbirth classes discuss what life will be like after the baby is born. They'll cover how to feed and bathe a baby, how to swaddle them, and give different ideas for sleep training. It can be beneficial to have your partner present for this information because they'll see that all of this care shouldn't fall on the new mother. Many people think a breast-feeding mother is all the baby needs for the first few weeks of their life, but in reality, both parents should spend time caring for and bonding with the baby. Your partner can better support you postpartum after learning the things taught in these classes!

Beyond significant events like doctor's appointments and childbirth classes, talk to your partner about what else they can do to support you

during pregnancy. Talk to them about helping out with the cooking and the cleaning. Even if they are busy with work and other things, they will want to support you in any way that they can. If you are having trouble exercising, eating healthy, or giving up coffee, ask your partner

to change some of their habits to match your new ones. Your partner

wants to be a big part of your pregnancy, and having them make the changes you are making will be extremely helpful. They can help keep you accountable and push you if you feel like giving up.

Besides physically being with you in a show of support, your partner can support you emotionally by making sure they're in tune with you and asking what you need. It can be hard to ask for help whether you're pregnant or not, but especially with your hormones making you emotional, asking for help can seem like a step too far! If your partner is paying attention to your needs, you'll feel more supported and less stressed throughout the pregnancy.

Physical affection varies from person to person. Some women want to be left alone because their body is changing so much they can hardly come to grips with it, much less invite someone else to touch them. Other women crave physical affection, being told they're beautiful, and having sex during pregnancy. No matter how you feel, you're fine—remember, there is no "normal." Just make sure your partner knows how you feel and supports you. It can be frustrating to have a partner cuddling you if you want to be left alone. On the other hand, it can be isolating and send you into a depression if you want to be touched and complimented, but your partner isn't giving you that.

Even if you don't want physical affection, your body might benefit from massages or foot rubs, so ask your partner if they're willing to do that for you. These actions can also boost you mentally and emotionally, so it might be worth the touch to get the all-around relaxing benefits of massage.

Though you're the person carrying the baby and going through so many physical, emotional, and mental changes, don't push all of the other responsibilities onto your partner. While it'd be nice for them to do as much as they can so you can rest and stay healthy, they might have personal stresses. Keeping an open line of communication during pregnancy is crucial. You don't want your partner to feel put-upon because they're taking over so many household tasks.

You might find that your partner has many of the same worries and anxieties about pregnancy, birth, and parenthood. Talking over these together can help ease your fears and strengthen your bond as partners and make you better parents. Be clear and specific with your partner about your current and future expectations for you and them. Let them tell you what they think will happen, so you both have the big picture of the possibilities of this journey.

If you're doing this alone, don't feel discouraged. Having a partner can be handy, but you can build up your own community while you're pregnant, even if you lack a family support system. Many hospitals and birthing centers arrange meet-ups and support groups for pregnant women. You can also find online support groups for the month your baby will be born so that you can compare experiences and milestones with women on the same timeline. You can also take prenatal yoga, exercise classes, or childbirth education to meet friends and build a support system.

After your baby is born, you can find support in breastfeeding organizations and meet-ups for new parents. Many areas also offer Mommy and Me Yoga and exercise classes to help you feel more at home in your new body. Since physical activity is so important during pregnancy, you'll want to keep up the habit even after giving birth.

3

TAKING CONTROL OF YOUR PHYSICAL HEALTH THROUGH EXERCISE

When your body is changing and your hormones are fluctuating, having to exercise on top of that might seem like too much to handle. The best thing to remember is how exercise will help you and the baby in the long run. You don't have to do 45 minutes of cardio to benefit from some movement in your life. Simply being active will boost your physical well-being, as well as your mental and emotional health. Even then, it's important to be in tune with your body and always be aware of how you feel. Don't overdo it! Just like everything else in pregnancy, exercise should be done in moderation.

Exercise is vital because it's a healthy habit that will positively affect you and your baby. When you feel good after exercising, you're more likely to decrease other unhealthy habits as a result. Exercising makes you feel healthy and boosts your serotonin levels so that you feel peaceful and calm afterward. Maintaining exercise and other healthy habits during pregnancy can help prevent complications and make childbirth and your postpartum experience easier to manage.

While many of your aches and pains during pregnancy are caused by your changing body and hormones, exercise can:

- help ease backaches
- promote muscle tone
- ease bloating and swelling
- prevent excessive weight gain
- boost your mood and energy levels

Exercises in later trimesters can help lower your risk of gestational diabetes, shorten the time of your labor, and reduce your risk of having a C-section.

Make sure you get your doctor's approval before exercising, and always slowly warm-up for the physical activity, drink plenty of water, and cool down to prevent any muscle pain. There are different exercises for each trimester, so make sure you're doing activities you're capable of, and always listen to your body!

ALL TRIMESTERS

It's recommended to get about 30 minutes of moderate-intensity exercise every day. Moderate intensity means you should still be able to carry on a conversation while you're exercising. Even if you're exercising alone, try to talk normally and make sure you're able to breathe and talk simultaneously. Struggling for breath while talking means you're working your body too hard. If you're pushing your body too much, you'll pull oxygen and blood flow away from your uterus and send it to the muscles you're working on instead.

Do not participate in contact sports or exercises that put you at risk of falling. You're always able to do cardiovascular and aerobic exercises throughout your pregnancy. These exercises include walking, jogging, swimming, and riding a stationary bike. You should avoid any activity that puts too much stress on your joints.

If you weren't big into exercising before pregnancy, don't be too intimidated to start! And don't jump right in with 30 minutes of exercise a day because you might strain your muscles. It's better to start with 10 minutes of movement a day, whether this is walking, gentle stretching, or another exercise that will ease your body into daily practice. Even low-impact exercise for 10 minutes a day will help you develop the habit so that you're making time for it and can ease your body into more involved activities over a few days.

Start adding five minutes of exercise to your daily limit after you feel comfortable with your 10 minutes of movement. Then add five more until you build up to 30 minutes a day. You can vary your activities each day, so you don't get bored doing the same thing. Changing up your exercises instead of sticking to a set routine will also keep your body guessing and help the activity impact your muscles more.

It might not seem like much, but even adding movement by taking the stairs instead of the elevator can help improve the health of you and your baby. Walking around a grocery store doesn't seem strenuous, but taking the long way to find each item will add quality movement to your routine.

If you were very active before pregnancy, your body is acclimated to that level of activity, so you can keep it up, for the most part. Make sure you're not doing anything that could harm you or the baby, and run your activities by your doctor beforehand.

You might have trouble holding yourself account- able if you're working out on your own, so consider pulling your partner into the activities. You might have friends who would like to walk with you and catch up. If you're still working, you might want to make time on your lunch break to walk around and get some fresh air, and you could ask a coworker to come with you.

If that's not enough motivation and interaction for you, look for prenatal exercise classes in your community. Prenatal yoga is a great way to exercise your body and stretch your muscles gently and prepare for childbirth. Plus, you'll meet plenty of other expecting mothers there, so you can broaden your social circle while you work out!

FIRST TRIMESTER

In your first trimester, you're probably adjusting to so many physical, emotional, mental, and hormonal changes that exercise is the last thing on your mind! But moving every day can help balance your hormones and make you feel better in the long run, so it's a great time to start exercising and setting healthy habits for the rest of your pregnancy.

You'll want to implement exercises that strengthen your core immediately. You want to make your spine as strong and flexible as possible while also making your abdominal muscles strong enough to support your stomach as it grows.

One such exercise is the pelvic curl. Lie on your back with your knees bent so your feet can rest flat on the ground. Position your knees to be about hip-width apart. Take a deep breath before you start, then tuck your pelvis so that you're pressing your spine into the floor as you exhale. Continue exhaling so that you feel like you're emptying your lungs as you roll your hips and lift your spine slowly from the impression you made. Once you reach your shoulder blades, inhale again and exhale as you push your body back down to the floor slowly, vertebra by vertebra. Doing this 15 times is a quality workout for beginners that can strengthen the core. For more experienced athletes, make the exercise more challenging by pressing your knees together instead of keeping them hip-width apart.

Strengthening your pelvic floor is also something you should start doing during the first trimester and keep up through your pregnancy. A strong pelvic floor can keep you from having urinary issues during pregnancy and beyond and keep your pelvic floor in shape for intercourse and giving birth.

One exercise to strengthen your pelvic floor is the pelvic brace. Lie on your back with your knees bent and held hip-width apart, just like you did with the pelvic curl. Keep your feet flat on the ground. Rest your back naturally on the ground; there should be a small space between the floor and your lower back. Take a deep breath, then contract all of your openings when you exhale. This is a Kegel contraction that works on muscles surrounding your urethra, vagina, and anus. Feel how your abdominal muscles work to perform this contraction, and try to pull those muscles in even more while you're contracting your other muscles. When you inhale, you can relax your contractions and abdominal muscles. On your next exhale, tighten all of the muscles again.

You can do 10 to 15 of these breaths and contractions to make up a set. You should do at least two sets a day to work those muscles. Once you feel what muscles are being worked, you might find yourself doing Kegels even as you sit at your desk at work or when you're binge-watching a show on the couch! You're doing something good to benefit your future self any time you work these muscles, so don't shy away from them.

Squats are another exercise you can easily do to strengthen your lower body and prepare you for childbirth. Squats also help strengthen your back, so you might have less pain as your belly grows during pregnancy.

You can do squats anywhere you are, but it's easier to get into the swing of the exercise by using a couch or a chair against the wall to practice. Stand in front of the couch or chair with your back facing the furniture. Put your feet flat on the floor, a little wider than hip-width apart, so you feel balanced. Start to squat like you're going to sit on the couch or chair, but as soon as your thighs touch the furniture, start lifting your body back up. Take it slow!

Lowering yourself down should take about five seconds, and bringing your body back up should take at least three. Making this motion too fast can strain your muscles.

To make squats easier and feel more natural, exhale as you squat down and inhale as you stand back up. Doing this exercise 15 or 20 times counts as a set, and you should do at least two sets a day to get the most out of the workout.

During your first trimester, you might also want to introduce some lightweight training into your exercise routine to strengthen your upper body. If you don't have weights, you can do kneeling push-ups to develop your biceps.

Lie on your stomach, then push yourself up to your hands and knees. Keep your knees as far apart as your hips, but slightly behind your hips so you'll have more weight to push up. Pull in your abs the way you did during the pelvic brace exercise and lower your chest to the floor while breathing in. Inhaling as you complete this part of the workout should allow you to really tighten your abdominal muscles. Exhale as you push your body back up into position; this gives you a burst of energy as you push against your weight.

These push-ups aren't too difficult, so even a beginner can start with 10 a day. As you increase your workout time to 30 minutes, you should be able to do at least 20 kneeling push-ups.

After you develop your biceps with this exercise, you might want to invest in some light hand weights if you don't already have any around. Five- or 10-pound weights on dumbbells can help you with bicep curls because you'll soon be carrying around a baby that weighs about that much!

For bicep curls, hold the weights and stand with your feet slightly wider than your hips, so you feel balanced. Keep your knees slightly bent, so you don't strain your joints. Exhale as you bend your elbows to bring the weights toward your shoulders slowly. Inhale as you ease the weights back down to your hips. Like squats, this is another exercise you don't want to do too quickly. You shouldn't lift the dumb-bells faster than three seconds and take at least five seconds to lower them back down.

Bicep curls can be done in sets of 10 or 15, and you should aim to do two sets each time you tackle this exercise.

Keep in mind that all of these exercises are just suggestions. You're adjusting to so much during the first trimester that you don't want to further exhaust yourself with your workouts. Adding in some sort of exercise along these lines will definitely help you throughout pregnancy and childbirth, so when you're feeling up to the workout, consider trying those outlined in this section.

SECOND TRIMESTER

After your first trimester, you shouldn't do any exercises that ask you to lie on your back. Your uterus is getting bigger, so you'll have to be a little more cautious about the physical activities you're doing. Luckily, most women experience a burst of energy in the second trimester, so you might be ready for a change of workout routine anyway!

At this stage, you don't want to do any exercises that have you jumping, running, or push you to exhaustion. Your health and your baby's health are critical, so exercise that isn't beneficial for both of you needs to be put on hold until you completely recover from childbirth.

The squats you started in the first trimester are one exercise that you should carry over into this one. You can vary your form a little by putting your legs closer together for narrow squats. You can even try to squat while balancing on one leg, as long as you feel stable enough not to fall over!

By the second trimester, you should be ready to progress from kneeling push-ups to incline push-ups. Instead of getting on your hands and knees, stay standing and face a low ledge or railing. Put your hands on the ledge or railing shoulder-width apart, so your weight feels supported. Step back, so you're doing a standing plank with your body in a diagonal line from your shoulders to your feet. Bend your elbows slowly, bringing your body closer to the railing you're leaning against, then straighten your arms to push your body back into a line.

Do these push-ups in sets of at least 10 at a time, and aim for two sets per day. Just like the kneeling push-ups, you should go slowly. This helps your muscles grow stronger because they hold you in set positions instead of quickly lowering and dropping your weight.

You can work to strengthen your core even more by expanding your muscle focus to your hips, lower back, gluteal, and calves. Making these muscles stronger will not only help you prevent aches and pains during pregnancy but will also help you stay strong as you start carrying around your newborn!

As your belly grows in your second trimester, your center of gravity will change. When you're adding new exercises into your routine, make sure you go slowly from the start and practice them to make sure you're aware of your body as you move. You don't want to put yourself at risk of falling during these exercises.

Because of this changing center of gravity, stretching your hip flexor muscles will help you be more in tune with your body as it grows.

Start by kneeling on the floor, then lift your left leg so your foot is flat on the floor and you're only half-kneeling. Keep your back straight as you stretch toward your left foot until you feel your right hip and thigh muscles activate. Hold for 30 seconds while you feel the stretch in the muscles on your right side. Do this motion three times each set before switching positions. Put your right foot flat and lunge to your right, so you feel the stretch in the muscles on your left side.

Another way to help balance your changing center of gravity is to stabilize your pelvic muscles and thighs. A side-lying leg lift can help strengthen these muscles. Lie on your right side and stack your knees on top of each other, slightly bent. Try raising your right hip off the floor so that there is a gap between your waist and the floor. Lifting your body in this way will level your pelvis. After creating a gap between your waist and the floor, straighten your left leg and move it slightly in front of the rest of your body. Angle your left foot's toes to the floor and feel your hip rotate to make this possible. Exhale slowly and count to three while you lift your leg, and inhale and count to three while you bring it back down. Make sure you're keeping the gap between the right side of your waist and the floor open.

This exercise works multiple muscles that will help you carry your pregnancy weight more evenly. Make the same motions up to 15 times per set, and do two sets per side of your body each day.

As your body changes during the second trimester, you know your baby is growing enough to cause these changes! That growing baby can put pressure on your diaphragm and ribs, but instead of sucking it up and living with that discomfort, you can do a mermaid stretch to ease the pain.

Sit on the floor with your legs folded so that your feet are pointing to the right side of your body like they're a singular mermaid tail. Keep your back straight as you raise your left arm straight up to the sky while inhaling a deep breath. When you're ready to exhale, bend your torso to the right as you let the air leave your body. As you stretch, you'll feel the muscles on the left side of your body. If you're feeling discomfort on a specific side of your body, do this stretch several times with that side of your body experiencing the impact from the exercise. Otherwise, do the exercise evenly on both sides of your body to get the most benefit and potentially prevent diaphragm pain in the second trimester.

THIRD TRIMESTER

During your third trimester, you might find your energy waning, but it's important to still work out as much as you can without completely exhausting yourself. Remember, after your first trimester, you shouldn't participate in any exercises that ask you to lie on your back. You might want to do something that allows you to lie down, but by now, your baby is so large that being on your back isn't good for either of you!

At this time, you've strengthened your body from the exercises you did throughout your first and second trimesters, so you can slow down slightly to focus on cardiovascular exercises. These will keep your abdominal strength up to help during birth and your postpartum period. It would be best to focus on walking, swimming, pelvic floor exercises, and movement using light hand weights.

As your pubic bone starts to shift to prepare for natural childbirth, keeping your legs too far apart will make the pain in this area worse. If you continue doing exercises from the second trimester, adjust them, so your legs aren't more than hip-width apart. If your lower back or pelvis hurts when you're doing tasks like walking or standing, you can wear a back brace to help redistribute your weight and support your muscles.

Some exercises you might want to do while comfortably standing include lifting weights to strengthen your arm muscles. Simple repetitive bicep curls or slowly bringing hand weights over your head can help develop the muscles you'll frequently use with your new baby.

If you have the opportunity to swim, this can be great exercise for your third trimester. Being in the water takes so much stress off of your joints that you can get a lot of activity without discomfort! You can find water aerobics classes to join or swim laps on your own—both methods will raise your heart rate.

During your third trimester, you can also benefit from yoga and Pilates. While these movements are appropriate throughout your entire pregnancy, you might especially benefit from them at the end as you prepare your body for childbirth. Since there aren't too many other exercises you can safely do at this point, yoga and Pilates can help you keep your body moving.

Yoga and Pilates both help you stretch your muscles, build up their strength, and safely expand your flexibility. Building these muscles can decrease your likelihood of back pain and help your body stay strong as the baby shifts in preparation for birth.

Prenatal yoga and Pilates classes also include exercises that strengthen your pelvic floor. We've already gone over some you can do independently, but it's nice to continue doing them in your third trimester by integrating them into a more extensive workout routine.

Since practicing these exercises gives you time to be calm and thoughtful, you can use focused breathing and mindfulness to calm your body and mind. These exercises can reduce stress and anxiety and decrease your chances of depression.

You can do two sessions of yoga or Pilates a week, but take a day off between them, so you don't push yourself too hard. Make sure you're staying hydrated and being mindful of your breathing. Remember that you should still be able to carry on a conversation while exercising. As your baby gets bigger, you might not be able to exercise as you once did and still be able to talk and breathe normally, so make sure you're aware of your limits. That includes your changing center of gravity as the baby grows.

If you're taking prenatal yoga or Pilates classes, every pose should be appropriate for you and your baby. If anything feels uncomfortable, adapt it to your ability, or don't do the pose. If you're watching videos online, make sure you remember not to do any poses that require you to lie on your back. Your baby's weight can push on your blood vessels and cut off circulation to you or the baby, causing you to feel faint and dizzy.

Drink water before and after you exercise and keep a bottle of water nearby if you start to feel dehydrated. Make sure you eat a small meal or snack before and after exercising to help combat any dizziness. Eating good foods can help give you energy for your work-out, so let's see what some of the best foods are for you and your growing baby.

4

TAKING CONTROL OF YOUR PHYSICAL HEALTH THROUGH YOUR DIET

It's essential to eat enough during your pregnancy to satisfy both you and your baby, but you'll only need to eat about 300 extra calories a day to nourish you both. The important thing is that you're eating the right foods. Your doctor might tell you that your baby will get the nutrition they need no matter what, so shift your focus to eating a balanced diet that will keep you both healthy.

Just like a lack of moderate exercise can negatively impact your baby's health, eating an unhealthy diet can also put them at a disadvantage before they're born. Eating a selection of foods from the five food groups will give you a good start to having a healthy diet. You can also supplement your diet with vitamins and other nutrients.

WHAT TO AVOID

Before we get to the good stuff, let's take a look at foods you should avoid. First and foremost is alcohol. It's common sense, and most women know this, but you might not think about abstaining until you find yourself in a situation where everyone else is drinking, and you reach for one out of habit. Even a small amount of alcohol can harm your unborn baby, so you shouldn't drink at all during your pregnancy and while you're breastfeeding.

You want to limit your sugar intake, so it's best to avoid chocolate, cookies, desserts, pastries, and soft drinks. You might have a craving for something sweet, but fruit can satisfy your sweet tooth while also delivering nutrients to you and your baby. All of the previously mentioned foods also offer little nutritional goodness, so you should avoid them.

Foods that are high in fat should also be eaten in moderation. You should eat foods that are high in polyunsaturated or monounsaturated fats instead of eating a lot of butter, cream, oil, and salad dressing. This doesn't mean you're sacrificing taste! You can use certain oils and spreads for salads and sandwiches, as well as nut butters and avocados.

Salt is another seasoning you should limit. Try not to use much when you're cooking, and don't add any to your meal when you're ready to eat. Salt can raise your blood pressure and cause heart problems. Your hormones and changing body can already lead to swelling in your face, hands, ankles, and feet, and eating too much salt will exacerbate this.

Be extra cautious in ensuring your food is safe to eat. Wash all fruits and vegetables before you eat them, so you're removing all traces of soil from the food. Soil can contain a parasite called toxoplasma, which can harm your baby.

Wash everything very carefully when you're cooking raw meat. You don't want to accidentally use a fork that has touched raw chicken because it can make you sick from listeria and salmonella. Ensure you cook your meat all the way through before you eat it, and try to eat it when it's as hot as possible.

Lastly, store your foods safely. Raw food should be in separate containers than ready-to-eat foods to prevent contamination. This is especially important when storing meat! Store it in its own container to avoid contaminating other foods with salmonella, E. Coli, or campylobacter.

Caffeine should also be limited when you're pregnant. Some women find it easier to quit cold turkey than to have a little, so your approach will be personal. You should only have about 200 milligrams of caffeine each day, which is the equivalent of one 12-ounce cup of coffee. Even after the baby is born, you shouldn't have more than two cups of coffee a day if you're breastfeeding.

This limit is because caffeine increases your blood pressure and heart rate and passes through the placenta to your baby. If caffeine makes you feel jittery and anxious, you definitely don't want to cause your baby to feel this way!

THE FIVE FOOD GROUPS

The five food groups are fruits, vegetables, grains, protein, and dairy. You should eat foods from all five groups every day, though the recommended servings vary. Each food group has nutrients your body needs that will impact your health in different ways.

As you explore your food choices during pregnancy, you might find that they have added benefits for you. Some women love to eat almonds to stave off their nausea. Other women love greens when they need to feel energized and focus.

Different foods can impact you in different ways, so as long as you're getting adequate amounts in your daily diet, you'll discover the benefits they may have on you in ways beyond general health!

Fruit

You should aim to eat two cups of fruit a day, with a focus on whole fruits. These fruits can be fresh, frozen, canned, or dried. Fruit juice can also help you reach your recommended servings as long as it does not have too much added sugar.

Fresh fruit has just enough natural sugar that it can be a great snack when you're feeling tired because the sugar will energize you. Many fruits include vitamins you need during pregnancy, so eating them will do more than satisfy your sugar craving. The best fruits to eat during pregnancy are:

- apples
- oranges
- apricots
- bananas
- grapes

- berries
- pears
- mangoes
- guava
- pomegranates
- avocados

These fruits have nutrients that keep you healthy and allow your baby to grow. Many of these vitamins will help boost your immune system, so you're less likely to get sick during pregnancy. That immunity will stimulate your baby's budding system as well! Eating enough fruit during pregnancy can supply your baby with enough iron to prevent anemia and enough calcium to help their bones grow strong. Of course, you'll benefit from the iron and calcium too.

While all of these fruits will give you excellent health during pregnancy, there are a few to spotlight for their unique features. Apples reduce the possibility of your baby developing asthma and allergies over time, so this might be a fruit you want to keep on hand for daily snacking (Willers et al., 2007).

Oranges are an especially key fruit to eat unless you have a strong aversion to them. They are so juicy that they help you stay hydrated. Oranges are chock full of vitamin C that facilitates iron absorption and can prevent cell damage, and help them heal. Best yet, they include folate, which can prevent neural tube defects. Neural tube defects can cause problems with your baby's brain and spinal cord, so eating oranges is a great way to get the nutrients you need to prevent that.

Bananas might be your favorite fruit during your first trimester. They're full of vitamins, fiber, and potassium. Vitamin B-6, in particular, has been shown to relieve nausea in pregnant women, so grabbing a banana as a healthy snack can have multiple benefits for you and your baby!

Fresh fruit is the best choice if you have access to it, but even dried fruit is packed with vitamins, nutrients, and fiber. If you're choosing dried fruit instead of fresh, change your portion size accordingly. You'll need to eat less dried fruit because they have been dehydrated, so you're getting the same nutrients from a smaller package. Try to balance dried fruit with fresh fruit, so you're still getting the water content that helps aid digestion.

Vegetables

You should eat two and a half cups of veggies a day. They can be fresh or frozen, but you should avoid canned vegetables whenever possible. You'll get more nutrients out of vegetables that are in season. Make sure to eat a variety of vegetables, including dark green, red, and orange veggies. Varying your vegetables will also give you more options in terms of the meals you're making, so try not to get stuck on one type.

Eating vegetables during pregnancy can help prevent gestational diabetes and low birth weight. They're also high in vitamins and fiber, so they'll help your weight gain stay moderate and healthy. Vegetables are high in beta carotene, which will help your baby develop their immune system and internal tissues, as well as improve their eyesight.

Just like with some fruits, vegetables have vitamin C and folic acid. Vitamin C helps your baby strengthen their teeth and bones, while folic acid helps prevent neural tube defects. Potassium is also found in vegetables and will help both you and your baby regulate your blood pressure.

The best vegetables to eat when you're pregnant include:

- tomatoes
- bell peppers
- broccoli
- green peas
- dark leafy greens
- sweet potatoes
- beetroot
- parsley

You can eat veggies raw or cooked, so if you like the taste of any from this list, eat up! If you prefer to hide your vegetables in other dishes, you can add seasonings and roast several of these vegetables, like bell peppers and sweet potatoes. You can also mix them all into a stir fry and add sauce to taste. Making vegetable soup is a great way to get your daily servings, and you can make a big batch at once, so you have leftovers for later.

While you can eat dark leafy greens and create your own salad, bagged salad or salad bars are not great choices for your vegetables during pregnancy. Raw sprouts might seem like a healthy choice, but they are also likely to expose you to bacteria that can harm your growing baby. Listeria is a bacteria that can grow on refrigerated foods; it can be killed by cooking, but of course, you won't cook a bag of ready-made salad or sprouts; therefore, it's best to avoid those until you give birth.

If you're not a vegetable fan typically, don't be afraid to try new foods during pregnancy. Knowing how good the vegetables are for you might help you enjoy them more. Plus, your tastes are changing, so you might find that you like a vegetable you had never appreciated before!

Grains/Starches

Eating grains is crucial because they are full of nutrients like iron, magnesium, and selenium. They have plenty of B vitamins that help your baby grow, as well as help keep your placenta healthy. You should eat six ounces of grains and starch a day, prioritizing whole grains.

Whole grains have the most vitamins and nutrients, and the label of any food item will tell you if it's made with whole grains. If the package isn't stamped to let you know it contains whole grains, grains are usually listed first on the ingredients list. Whole wheat bread and brown rice are two good examples of whole grains that give you plenty of nutrients.

If a food says it uses "refined" or "enriched" grains, it won't be as healthy for you and your growing baby.

Try to find whole-grain items whenever possible. In addition to all of the nutrients they contain, they also have plenty of fiber. Fiber will help with digestion, as well as prevent constipation and hemorrhoids.

Examples of grains to eat during pregnancy include:

- whole wheat
- corn
- rice
- oats
- barley

Whole wheat bread, whole wheat bagels, and cornbread are excellent foods to eat during pregnancy. You can also eat oatmeal, whole-grain cereal, or whole-grain waffles for breakfast. You can cook brown rice or wild rice as a side with your dinner and add sauce or seasonings for taste. You can even eat three cups of popcorn as a snack to consume your daily grains; just skip the butter and salt!

If you feel like you're not getting enough grains in your diet, see what other alternatives your store might have in stock. Some noodles are made from whole grains, so you could use those for spaghetti or pasta sides to get some extra servings in. You can also use whole-grain flour in your baked goods to get the benefit of grain.

Protein

Protein is made of amino acids that are also in your body's cells. Proteins create muscles, bones, skin, and hair. Eating protein during your pregnancy will help build your baby's cells, especially during the second and third trimesters when your baby is growing fast to prepare for birth.

Exactly how much protein you need will vary depending on your weight, so check with your doctor for specifics. The general guidelines are to eat five and a half ounces of protein every day while making sure you're mixing up the types of protein. Even if you're craving chicken, don't eat it too many days in a row. Mix up your protein intake to include other lean meats, nuts, beans, and peas.

You're more than likely already getting enough protein in your daily diet, so you don't need to consume too much more when you're pregnant. If you're having trouble eating enough protein every day, don't stress about it. Aim to eat an average of the correct amount each week, which might be an easier way to get the benefits you need from protein.

Usually, you could tell if you're not getting enough protein in your diet because you'd feel exhausted, have muscle fatigue, and notice fluid retention. Still, those traits can be common during any stage of pregnancy, so you might not know you're missing out. If you're losing weight instead of gaining it or have frequent infections, you should try to increase your protein intake and see if that helps improve your health.

Good sources of protein include:

- lean meat
- chicken
- fish
- eggs
- beans
- milk
- cheese
- yogurt
- tofu

Eggs, cheese, and yogurt are great ways to get protein in the morning or as a snack. Meats, fish, beans, and tofu can create a variety of meals for lunches and dinners to ensure you're getting protein at every meal. Remember, snacking on nuts or peanut butter will also give you a helping of protein in a convenient snack. You can toss various nuts and dried fruits together to make your own trail mix to snack on throughout the day. This is a great way to get protein and boost your energy between meals.

Keep in mind that not all fish is safe to consume during pregnancy. Salmon is ideal because it is high in omega-3 fatty acids that promote your baby's brain development. Light tuna is also a quick and easy choice for making lunches, as long as you don't eat more than 12 ounces per week. You can also eat trout, tilapia, and shrimp when you're pregnant. Avoid fish that is high in mercury or contaminated with pollutants. This includes eating sushi made with raw fish or any that has high mercury levels. You might want to look for a roll that is made with imitation crab meat if you're really craving sushi!

Chicken and turkey are excellent choices for protein if you eat meat. You can pair them with so many different grains and vegetables to give you a well-rounded lunch or dinner. You can substitute ground turkey for ground beef in any recipe, so you're making a healthier choice in terms of fat.

Your meat choices aren't limited to chicken and turkey; other lean meats like lean beef, pork, or lamb make great dinners. You can pair them with a side or use them as an ingredient in a soup, salad, noodle dish, or casserole. Beans can be a great side or incorporated into vegetable soup. You can even make black bean burgers if you're a vegetarian—or if you just want to try a different kind of burger!

Eggs are so versatile that you can eat a serving of them per day and not have to worry about your overall protein intake. You can scramble eggs or make an omelet for breakfast, eat a hardboiled egg plain or cut it onto a salad, or even top a turkey burger with a fried egg!

Dairy

We already mentioned a few dairy items in the protein section—that's how important they are! Dairy supplies calcium, protein, and vitamin D that help your baby develop bones, teeth, heart, muscles, and nerves.

You should consume three cups of dairy a day. This doesn't have to be milk, but if you're drinking milk, make sure it's low-fat or fat-free. Dairy includes cheese, yogurt, and soy. The specific dairy products you choose to consume might depend on your weight; if you're underweight, full-fat dairy products can give you the calories you need to keep up your health.

Dairy can be easy to consume if you like to drink milk, eat cereal with milk for breakfasts or snacks, or like yogurt and cheese. You can use evaporated milk in place of regular milk in recipes because it has twice the calcium. This can be a great substitute in macaroni and cheese, mashed potatoes, smoothies, and any casserole that calls for milk.

You can use a yogurt base to make a tasty dip for all of the fresh fruits and vegetables you're eating. It's a different way to incorporate these foods into your diet, with the added bonus of dairy, instead of always serving them as sides for meals.

You can always add more cheese too! Eat an extra-cheesy grilled cheese sandwich using whole-grain bread. Add shredded cheese to the top of any casserole you're making. Cook macaroni and cheese so that it's even cheesier than before.

Keep in mind that you can't eat soft cheeses and cheeses made from unpasteurized milk while you're pregnant, though. These are more likely to have listeriosis, a bacteria that can make you ill. Unpasteurized milk can also contain listeriosis, so make sure you read the label before buying milk or a product made with milk.

Even if you're lactose intolerant, your body can still handle one cup of milk once a day, especially if you eat something else with the milk. You can also opt to buy lactose-reduced milk or split one glass of milk into four smaller servings, so it's easier to digest over time. Hard cheeses have the lowest lactose content out of dairy items, which might be a pleasant and tasty way to get the dairy you need. Talk to your doctor about how you can make sure you're getting enough dairy in your diet if you're lactose intolerant.

If you are struggling to eat the appropriate amount of any of these different food groups, try incorporating them into your meals differently. You could try blending up vegetables into a pasta sauce or make fruit smoothies. Sometimes switching up your usual routine can make it easier to maintain a healthy diet.

SUPPLEMENTS AND VITAMINS

If there are certain foods you can't eat, like the previously mentioned lactose, you might consider adding supplements to your diet. Consult your doctor before adding any supplements and vitamins to your diet with caution because some aren't safe for pregnancy. Your doctor might take a blood test at the beginning of your pregnancy to look for any nutrient deficiencies. If changing the way you eat isn't possible due to an intolerance, diet preference, or food allergies, they can recommend vitamins and supplements that are safe for pregnant women to fill in those nutritional gaps.

Prenatal Vitamins

The American College of Obstetricians and Gynecologists (ACOG) recommends that all pregnant women take prenatal vitamins and folic acid supplements. Some prenatal vitamins will include folic acid, so read the ingredients carefully and consult with your doctor to see if you need both.

Many adults take daily vitamins to ensure they're getting all of the nutrients they need in addition to their balanced diets. However, prenatal vitamins are specifically formulated to give pregnant women all of the nutrients their baby needs as it grows. Though the name "prenatal" sounds like it's something you'll only take during pregnancy, you can start taking these vitamins when you're trying to conceive and continue taking them while you're breastfeeding.

Prenatal vitamins alone aren't enough to replace a balanced diet, but they're effective at filling the gaps. They reduce the risk of preterm birth and preeclampsia, a birth complication that results in high blood pressure and dangerous delivery conditions.

If you're already taking prenatal vitamins, you might not need to take any other supplements to get the nutrients you need. If you already have one, show your doctor what you're taking so they'll know what else your growing baby needs. If you're not already taking a prenatal vitamin, your doctor will help you find the best one for your body.

Folic Acid

Folic acid is a synthetic form of folate, a B vitamin that plays a significant role in DNA synthesis and fetal development. Folate can be found naturally in foods like eggs, legumes, leafy greens, citrus foods, nuts, and seeds. With a balanced diet from the five food groups, you might be getting enough folate naturally.

If not, you can take a folic acid supplement. Taking a supplement is a great idea because it reduces the risk of your baby having neural tube defects, and there are no side effects linked to having too much folate in your system.

Iron

Since your body is making more blood during pregnancy, you might need more iron than you can produce. Iron is necessary to transport oxygen to your baby and keep your placenta healthy during pregnancy. If you're anemic, you might have a preterm delivery, suffer from maternal depression, and your baby is more likely to be anemic as well.

Prenatal vitamins usually contain enough iron for mom and baby, but if you need more, your doctor will let you know and help you find the right supplement to take. Ensure your doctor is involved in this process because taking an iron supplement if you're not deficient can cause constipation, nausea, and elevated hemoglobin levels.

Other Vitamins

Other vitamins you might consider including vitamin D, which will boost your immune system and increase your bone health. If you have a vitamin D deficiency, you're at risk for having a cesarean section, giving preterm birth, and passing along gestational diabetes. Your doctor can screen you to see if you have a vitamin D deficiency.

Magnesium is another mineral that will boost your immune system, so getting enough during pregnancy can keep you and your baby healthy. It also helps develop muscles and nerve function to reduce your risks of preterm birth and fetal growth problems.

Fish oil contains two essential fatty acids that will boost your baby's brain development. While studies have differed in their findings, it seems that fish oil helps improve your baby's brain and eyes and decreases your risk of depression. If you'd rather only take supplements with proven results, never fear! You'll get enough fish oil if you eat two or three servings of low-mercury fish a week like salmon, pollock, or sardines. If you're eating this seafood as part of your balanced diet, you'll most likely be getting enough fish oil naturally.

Probiotics are a supplement of living microorganisms that help aid your digestion and improve your gut health. They are safe to take as pills or as drinkable yogurt during pregnancy and reduce the risk of gestational diabetes and postpartum depression.

Supplements to Avoid

If you're taking prenatal vitamins, you'll already be getting enough vitamin A, so avoid taking a separate vitamin A supplement. Too much vitamin A can be harmful, and since it's a fat-soluble vitamin, your body stores the excess. This can lead to liver damage and congenital disabilities. Vitamin E is another fat-soluble vitamin that you'll get naturally with no need to take a supplement.

You can use herbal supplements as natural remedies for headaches, body pains, nausea, and more. These can be fine for yourself, but they might harm your baby. Think about all of the pills and supplements you usually take, and make sure your doctor knows everything you're taking. Many of these herbal supplements are okay to take during pregnancy as long as you're buying them from a reputable brand held to standards from the United States Pharmacopeia (USP).

Don't start taking any new supplements during pregnancy without discussing it with your doctor first. Remember, your doctor is there to help, so you should use their expertise to help keep your body in tip-top physical shape during pregnancy. Let your doctor know what supplements you were taking before you got pregnant so you can work together to decide if you should continue taking these or stop them until you've given birth and stopped breast-feeding.

FIVE TIPS TO HELP YOU TAKE CONTROL OF YOUR EMOTIONS

Just as important as your physical health during pregnancy is your emotional well-being. With all of the hormonal changes you're going through, keeping control of your emotions might seem nearly impossible! Thankfully, taking small steps and making time for yourself can help you stay in charge of your emotions before they get the best of you.

It might feel like you're riding a roller coaster throughout your pregnancy journey, and trying to control everything will make you feel better about what you're going through. However, some things will happen that you won't be able to control, so sometimes it's best to sit back and let yourself feel everything, even if it's painful or isolating. Trying to ignore your emotions or push past the hard parts can harm you more in the long run than allowing yourself to feel everything.

However, feeling your emotions doesn't mean you have to wallow in them, giving them the power to stress you out or depress you. It's possible to feel your emotions, acknowledge them, and move forward. Taking that element of mindfulness and applying it to your daily life can help you fully experience your entire pregnancy without allowing your emotions to take charge. Learning about mindfulness and practicing it during pregnancy can help you stay in control while tackling your fear of the unknown.

1. WRITE IN A JOURNAL

When you write in a journal, you're capturing your thoughts and putting them on the page so you can have them available to read later. Please note that this doesn't mean you *have* to read them later! Sometimes it's handy to get thoughts out of your mind by putting them on paper, so they're not constantly swirling through your head. But if you're genuinely writing things down to get them out of your mind, you might not want to revisit them later! So you don't have to write in your journal with the intent to read it later, nor do you have to share these pages with anyone else.

If you're writing to get your thoughts onto paper, you might choose to write free form, which means you're sitting down with a pen and your journal and writing with no set goal or purpose in mind. This can help you feel better emotionally because you're letting everything pour out. Sometimes it's easier to let these thoughts and emotions out on the page instead of telling anyone around you. Also, just because you're writing something down doesn't mean you can't talk about it with someone! Writing things down can help you gather and organize your thoughts, so you feel more prepared for deeper conversations.

Journaling for mental health is a very worthwhile activity, but if you want to keep a journal and don't know what to write about, you don't need to skip this step! Using prompts as you journal can help keep your thoughts more focused on specific topics.

When you use prompts, you are finding questions that give you time to reflect. These prompts can help you think about specific topics you might have pushed to the back of your mind so that you have more time and energy for everything else each day, especially on days when your growing baby is exhausting you. You might feel so distracted by everything you have to do each day that you don't have time to focus your thoughts or process your emotions, and journaling can help you accomplish that.

If you feel stuck, try starting with:

- "Today, I feel…"
- "Right now, I want…"
- "I've been thinking…"
- "I am grateful for…"
- "_____ made me laugh today."
- "Today, my partner and I…"
- "I need help with…"

If you want to keep a pregnancy journal that you might like to share with your baby one day, you can use prompts customized to your journey.

- What is your best pregnancy memory so far?
- What are you excited about in terms of becoming a parent?

- What's something that will change from your old life when you become a parent?
- What's one trait you know you want to have as a parent?
- What's a memory from your parents that you would like to share with your child?
- What's your strongest memory from childhood that you'd share with your own child?
- What are three life lessons you learned that you want your child to know?

Writing can also help you heal after something traumatic. When you're pregnant, sometimes even your thoughts can feel traumatic! You might want to take time to process what you went through, waiting for prenatal test results, or discovering some illnesses in your family history. You might find that writing about these events is enough to help you feel more in control of the situation, but it's also okay to look at your writing and realize you need more help processing things.

Sometimes writing about your thoughts and emotions will help you let them go. Instead of continually stressing over the same thing, you might be able to write them and feel them a little less strongly, almost as if you're sharing your worries with someone else. You might find that, after writing about your emotions, you were overreacting over something minor, and you can let it go. Or you might find that an emotion you've been feeling was covering an underlying trauma and inspires you to seek help.

No matter what, keeping a journal can help you organize your thoughts and gain perspective. Pregnancy passes in such a blur that you might not remember what you felt at your last check-up when it's time for the next. If you've been writing down your thoughts and emotions, you can flip back to that day in your journal and remember what happened. You can also read back over things you wrote at the beginning of your pregnancy and see how much your thoughts and emotions have changed as your pregnancy progressed!

If you make journaling a ritual, you might find that you look forward to sitting down with a pen and notebook and spending a little time with your thoughts. There is so much hustle and bustle on an average day, and that is accelerated and compounded during pregnancy! Focusing on preparing your life for your new baby and working on your relationship with your partner can have you feeling left behind. Taking time to journal just for the sake of it—for release, not perfection—can help you feel like you're getting in touch with yourself for at least a few minutes each day.

And that's the best thing about journaling! It doesn't have to be a big hurrah. You can use any pen and any notebook. Find a quiet place to think at a time of day when you're not stressed, thinking of what else you should be doing. Carve this time out for yourself. Don't worry about what you're writing down, how emotional you're being, or how your handwriting looks. This is for you and you only. And you don't have to look at it ever again once you get your thoughts on paper.

If you give journaling a try and find yourself stuck for something to write about, don't give up. Give yourself a week or two of dedicated time to really try journaling before you decide you don't get anything out of it. You might be surprised how much it helps you after just a few sessions.

2. KEEP OPEN COMMUNICATION

In chapter two, we talked about how your partner can support you throughout your pregnancy. The focus was primarily on how they can take some stress and housework off your plate, so you're freer to take care of your changing body and growing baby. However, it's essential to keep open communication with your partner, so you both feel supported and prepared for what's to come.

When you write in your journal, you're doing that for yourself. You're giving yourself time to be alone and get in touch with your thoughts and emotions. It's important not to lose yourself during pregnancy because feeling lost and left behind contributes to feelings of depression and anxiety. Communicating with your partner is equally important, so neither of you feels left out in your relationship and your parenthood journey.

It can be tough to keep your relationship a priority when you have so many significant family changes coming at you in a few short months. It makes sense that you want to talk about the baby more than anything and prepare your house and life for the bundle of joy that's on the way, but you don't want to risk your relationship.

You might feel like you are burdening your partner with your emotions, but sharing your feelings can help them open up as well. They might feel closer to you because they're having similar thoughts but were too scared to bring them up with you. They might have solutions or different ways of thinking about similar problems, so together you can talk about the issues and help each other feel better. You will be amazed at how relieved you can feel when you open up the lines of communication.

It can be hard to understand your partner at this time because you're going through so much, and they seem to be staying the same. Your body is visibly changing, sure, but your thoughts, emotions, and hormones are changing on the inside, and your partner has no idea what you're going through. Even if you talk to them and try to describe what you're feeling, they can't really understand what you're going through. It can be easy, at that moment, to get angry with your partner because of what you're going through. Give your partner the benefit of the doubt and assume they are doing their best to understand and help you. You want to try and tell them what you're going through because they'll never experience it. For all the ups and downs you're experiencing, your body is doing something so amazing and awe-inspiring that your partner might feel left out.

If both you and your partner feel like you can talk about anything together, your relationship will benefit, and you'll feel so much less stress throughout your pregnancy. Of course, you'll still get mad at your partner because no one can do everything right, and your hormones are going up and down so much that having some extreme emotional reactions is bound to happen. However, if you're already more in touch with your own emotions through journaling, you'll be more likely to share those feelings with your partner so you can work together to move forward as parents being the strongest partners you can be.

3. DON'T BE AFRAID TO ASK FOR HELP

While you're working on being open with your partner, push yourself to ask for help when you need it, or even sometimes when you don't! It can be easy to feel like you need to be the one doing everything, but sometimes letting someone else do a task for you will not only give you a chance to relax, but it will make that person feel like they're doing something good for you. Remember, you want to build a community and a support system during your pregnancy so your child will grow up surrounded by love. Sometimes it's worth letting people help even when you know you're capable of doing a task yourself.

On the other hand, there are times when you know you can't do something on your own, and you shouldn't have to. It can be hard to ask for help; I think more people struggle with this than they'd care to admit. When you're pregnant and dealing with the hormones, emotions, and overall toll on your body, you might feel like you're incapable of doing one more thing. You might dissolve into a pile of tears because you know you need to complete certain tasks, but you just can't do it. Ask for help! If you feel like it's too much to ask your parents, in-laws, or neighbors for help, tell your partner what you need and let them help you, or find someone who can. This is where that open line of communication can save you some days. Being able to honestly tell your partner that you absolutely can't do one more thing can be a lifesaver.

You can open up lines of communication with other people by asking them for help before you need it. Maybe your mom makes the best enchilada casserole, so you can ask her to make you one to freeze before the baby's born. She'll understand that you're asking for help by having food ready after giving birth and might prepare several food items for you to stock up on. Or maybe knowing she can help in that way will help both of you think of other ways she can help in the meantime.

Never feel bad for asking for help, period. But especially when you need to do something that a pregnant woman can't do, like changing cat litter or climbing a ladder. No one will feel put-upon if a pregnant woman asks them for help and genuinely needs it. Once you start asking for help with the tasks you absolutely can't do, you might find it's easier to ask for help with other tasks.

If you're feeling exhausted and need a nap, don't push yourself to make dinner and clean the house before your partner gets home. They'll understand that you needed to rest more than you needed to have dinner on the table by the time they got home.

Asking for help can be challenging, but you should feel comfortable asking your partner for help with various tasks. Maybe the teenager next door can start taking the dog for a walk twice a day, and you can have your partner pick up take-out a couple of nights a week to cut down on cooking duties. Maybe a neighbor running an errand can pick up something for you on the way so you can stay home and nap instead of going to a store when you're feeling drained. It can be hard to ask, but once you look at the tasks you need to do each day and process who can help you handle them, you'll feel more prepared to ask for help, and the stress will ease off of your shoulders as a result. You will be surprised at how many people are willing to help you if you ask.

4. BE PREPARED FOR WHAT IS TO COME

Reading this book shows that you want to prepare yourself for pregnancy and parenthood, so you're already on a great path! You're taking steps to inform yourself, so you know what to expect while you're pregnant. You're learning what you can do to best prepare yourself, physically and mentally, for parenthood. You're taking care of your body by eating a healthy, balanced diet. You're taking care of your mind by realizing your emotions might be out of your control sometimes, but you can still process them in a way that makes them beneficial for you.

The baby is coming whether you're ready or not, so take advantage of the nine months to prepare your home for the baby. You can childproof your house while you're pregnant, so you and your partner get used to the changes. Putting special plugs in electrical outlets can help keep your child safe once they're toddling around independently. Installing childproof latches on kitchen cabinets will also keep your baby safe, but you might as well put them on now while you have time so that you can feel prepared.

Preparing for the baby doesn't always have to be serious, like childproofing your house. It can be fun, like painting the spare room and turning it into a nursery. You get to pick colors and themes and buy blankets that will cover your baby when you bring them home! You can research cribs, strollers, and car seats and buy what seems best for your family. You can take time to discuss names, nicknames and decide what type of baby announcement you'll send. You'll get to share the excitement with friends and family in terms of baby showers and giving them updates about doctor's appointments. There are so many ways to be prepared for your baby, so make sure you take time to enjoy it all. The key is to make this a joyful process. Don't stress over the little things and enjoy all the little things you can do to prepare for your baby.

5. TAKE TIME TO PROCESS YOUR EMOTIONS

It might sound cliche to process your emotions, but the truth is that many people don't take the time to do this. There's a difference between feeling an emotion and getting down to the root cause of it. You can feel an emotion without reflecting on why it made you feel a certain way. Taking time to process your emotions during pregnancy can help you feel in control of your feelings even when your hormones are raging.

Sometimes, just feeling emotions means you let them drown you. You might feel stuck in an inevitable cycle and not be able to remember how you used to feel or see a way out of what you're feeling now. Sometimes, you might not even allow yourself to feel emotions. If something seems negative or if you feel too busy, you might push your emotions aside. Letting your emotions drown you and pushing them aside are both detrimental to your overall well-being. Not taking the time to nurture your emotional side can lead to mental and physical problems. Ignoring your feelings or letting them rule your life can lead to making bad choices in terms of food, alcohol, unhealthy habits, and damaging relationships by lashing out and being angry.

Being pregnant will most likely amplify your emotions. It can be scary to sit with any negative feelings because you don't want to wallow in sadness or anxiety. But trying to feel positive all of the time is detrimental, too.

There's no reason to feel ashamed of however you're dealing with your emotions now. We're never really taught how to handle emotions; as children, we're often told to calm down and stay quiet instead of feeling our emotions. If you've gone to therapy, your counselor might have given you some ways to work through your emotions, but not everyone has that chance. Instead of drowning in your emotions—positive or negative!—learn how to process them so they can benefit you.

Emotions can be boiled down to five general topics: fear, anger, sadness, disgust, and joy. We experience these emotions because they result in the strongest reactions that benefit us in terms of fight or flight and survival. This shows that emotions are just a gut reaction to something that happens and can benefit from being mentally processed, so we better understand them.

While people often use the words emotions and feelings interchangeably, emotions are actually the broad categories mentioned above, and feelings fall under those bigger groups. We have five types of emotions but countless feelings under those giant umbrellas. Feelings are subjective, which is why some people react utterly opposite to the same trigger.

Time can influence feelings after you experience an emotion. You might also feel a certain way because of how you reacted to an emotion since those reactions are largely involuntary. Feelings give you space and distance to process emotions so you can learn from your mistakes. You might react differently to an emotion next time or try to avoid being put in that situation again in the first place.

Since being in touch with your feelings will help you learn from your mistakes and move forward in life positively, repressing your feelings can be damaging in the long run. If you never learn from what you've experienced, you might find yourself locked in a spiral of overwhelming negative emotions.

To take some of the pressure off of your feelings, remember that feelings are neutral as they are. The weight and value we assign to them are what makes them good or bad. So if you're worried about being overwhelmed by too many emotions, know that you can take a step back and look at your feelings from the outside to understand what they're telling you before you process them on a more personal level.

The basic foundation of processing your emotions is identifying what you're feeling, analyzing why you felt that way, and deciding how to handle your feelings by coping with them or resolving any issue you might have control over.

Sounds easy enough, right? Well, some people aren't aware of the subconscious ways they avoid feelings. Everyone has defense mechanisms in place to protect themselves from harmful emotions and situations. This doesn't mean you're experiencing a feeling and willingly turning a blind eye to it; you might not even realize you're doing it! Defense mechanisms can be ingrained in you from childhood, and it can be hard to acknowledge them and work to break them down. Luckily, you can process your feelings even if you have defense mechanisms in place.

Being mindful is the key to processing your emotions. Mindfulness is a way of thinking that lets you feel and experience every moment of your day without assigning judgment to it. When you judge yourself, and what you're feeling, you're making it harder to pull yourself through the experience. You're analyzing things while you're still in the middle of them instead of waiting until you're past them to assess your reaction.

Mindfulness also helps you get through tough times by giving yourself the space to feel while staying calm. Mindfulness and meditation can go hand in hand, but you don't have to meditate to benefit from taking a few quiet moments for yourself. Many people pair mindfulness with breathing exercises because it helps calm their emotions. The easiest breathing exercise to remember is the 4-7-8 breathing method. Inhale through your nose while counting to four. Hold your breath while you count to seven. Exhale through your mouth for eight beats. Do this as many times as you need until your body starts to calm down. As your body calms down, so will your emotions.

Being mindful also goes hand in hand with keeping a journal, and you may find that you like to link the two activities. Taking time to write about what you're feeling can help you acknowledge the emotions as you're going through them, then give you something to look back on once you've given yourself a little space.

Processing your emotions doesn't have to be a solitary endeavor. You can always share your feelings with your partner or other close friends and family members. They're ready to support you, and that includes listening to your feelings and validating you. Outside support can also help keep you grounded, so you don't feel overwhelmed by your emotions. These people know you and can help put your feelings into perspective.

While processing your emotions is usually done after you experience them, there are ways to calm yourself down in the moment. Being mindful is a great way, or by counting your breaths to soothe any overwhelming feelings. You might also choose to label your feelings as you experience them. Sometimes, taking a step back and saying, "I'm feeling angry," can help you realize what you're feeling and understand why you might not need to continue interacting with someone at that moment.

You might find that different approaches work better for you at different times. It's okay to have a wide range of ways to cope with your emotions! Staying mentally positive might also help you process your emotions during pregnancy.

6

ELEVEN TIPS ON STAYING MENTALLY POSITIVE DURING PREGNANCY

Hormones and stress can try to do their worst during pregnancy to make you feel anxious and depressed, but there are simple ways you can work to stay positive. Since worries and negative thoughts can be detrimental to your mental and physical health, you want to do all you can to stay positive for your baby.

If you're not naturally a chipper person, the weight of all of these life changes and hormones can make it even harder for you to feel happy. Then you feel bad that you're not feeling happy because who wouldn't be happy when they're about to become a mother? It can be a vicious cycle! Rest assured, whether you're a naturally optimistic person or not, you can take charge of different aspects of your life to stay mentally positive.

1. TAKE IT A DAY AT A TIME

Think of some of the worries you've had during pregnancy. Wondering what type of mother you'll be or imagining how your relationship with your partner might change after a few weeks of sleepless nights. You might worry about money and how expensive it will be to raise a child and send them to college.

What do all of these worries have in common? They're in the future! Instead of worrying about things that are far away, focus on what's going on right now. You don't need to think about what you're going to eat when you go out with friends next week; instead, focus on eating good food today. Don't worry about what labor will feel like; focus on taking a walk and doing some exercises right now to better prepare yourself for giving birth.

If you shift your focus from worries in the future to what you can do right now, you'll start to feel more in control of your body and your baby. Know that every step you take throughout your pregnancy is a way to move forward into a positive lifestyle. Eating right will keep your body healthy, which will impact your baby's health as well. Exercising will prime your body for giving birth, so you won't have a hard time with labor.

Mindfulness will help you take things one day at a time and stay in the moment as well. If you feel like future worries are overwhelming you, stop and breathe. Count your breaths and feel the air move in and out of your body. Focus on what you're feeling in the moment as your breaths calm you. Then, shift your thoughts, so you're not thinking of the future anymore. Instead, focus on what you're thinking and feeling right now. Let thoughts come and go in your mind, and don't grab onto anything in particular. Don't scold yourself for any thoughts; just let them float through your brain. When you finish this exercise, you'll feel calm and energized, and ready to focus on what's in your grasp today.

2. MAINTAIN A HEALTHY LIFESTYLE

You've learned a lot of tips about how to lead a healthy lifestyle while pregnant. Sometimes, it can seem too overwhelming to prepare a healthy meal or exercise for 30 minutes, but remember all of the benefits of a balanced diet and movement! Your baby will thank you for it. And your body will thank you also. It's easier to keep these healthy habits up after pregnancy if you've been doing them for several months, and your body will adapt easier postpartum.

A healthy lifestyle goes beyond just keeping your body in shape. Everything you consume will indeed filter through to the baby, so that's reason enough to eat right and exercise. But the serotonin released from exercise will also reach your baby, so when you feel good, your baby feels good.

The food you eat also greatly impacts your mood and energy levels. Even if you feel consumed by worries and none of the other methods on this list are helping you, food can always help you feel better. When you're eating healthy, you don't have to wait until the baby is born to see the results of your healthy lifestyle—you're benefiting from it instantly!

3. PREPARE FOR THE BABY'S ARRIVAL

It's almost impossible to feel down in the dumps when you're getting ready for your baby's arrival. Nesting vibes are real, and when you feel them, it's best to go with the flow. Get excited about preparing the baby's room, whether you're painting a new space or making a dedicated area for them in your own room.

Feeling productive while you're nesting can also help you feel more in control of all of the uncertainties on the horizon. Instead of worrying about what's to come, you know you're able to wash your baby's clothes and fold them into the dresser drawers. You can get diapers ready on the changing table and make sure you have the ointments and wipes needed. You can hang a mobile over the crib and position the glider just so.

It can be a lot of fun to let yourself get swept up in color swatches and nursery themes. Some people may think this is frivolous, but don't let them get to you. It's necessary to prepare for your baby's arrival, and being consumed by such a task will help you feel productive. It will also help you feel connected to your baby. You're preparing a special space just for them, so it's nearly impossible not to feel love blooming in your heart as you do so.

Preparing in advance for the baby's arrival also lets you take stock of all you have. You might realize that you have plenty of newborn onesies but no three-month clothes that are warm enough for the change of seasons. You can go shopping yourself, make an event of it with your partner or a friend, or add these items to your baby registry, so others will know what you need.

4. TAKE TIME FOR YOURSELF

With so much at stake during pregnancy, it can feel like too much to take time for yourself. Your life is changing, and you have so much to accomplish before the baby arrives, so you might feel like you're on a time crunch. But think about all that is going on in terms of your hormones, emotions, and changing body! This is the perfect time to pamper yourself because anything that makes you feel happier and more relaxed will also positively influence your baby.

You might enjoy getting manicures and pedicures to feel pretty while you're pregnant or trying a new hairstyle. You can also get massages and do some spa treatments, but make sure everything is safe for pregnancy. For example, you don't want a massage that requires you to lie on your stomach because that's not safe for babies. Many massage employees know about pressure points that can inspire labor and will avoid those as well. You won't want to sit in a sauna or a hot tub in terms of the spa because that heat won't be safe for you or the baby, but other treatments can help you relax.

You don't necessarily have to go somewhere to pamper yourself. You might want to go out for dinner or even order your favorite meal and eat it in the comfort of your own home. You might want to relax in the bathtub with some aromatherapy. You might just want an hour alone every evening to just be alone or read a book in silence. Whatever you like to do, make sure it's relaxing and that you're allowing yourself this time without feeling guilty. You're going to be so busy and sleep-deprived once the baby arrives that you need to soak up this solitude while you can!

5. FOCUS ON WHAT YOU CAN CONTROL

It can be easy to become overwhelmed with worries, but it's essential to be realistic with yourself and admit that there are some things you can't control. This can be hard to accept when it comes to your baby's life, but all you can do is manage the things that are under your control.

Luckily, you're taking significant steps towards this goal by reading this book, eating a balanced diet, and doing exercises that will keep you and your baby healthy. It might not seem like much, but while you're doing these things, each action is giving you broader results than you realize. The exercises in this book, for instance, not only keep you active and healthy during pregnancy but also help prepare your body for childbirth.

Preparing a birth plan can be especially beneficial for your mental and emotional health, but don't worry too much about controlling every aspect of childbirth. Your body and medical team will know the best way to safely bring your baby into the world. It can be disappointing when what actually happens differs from your ideal birth plan, but it's not the end of the world. As long as you get to hold your newborn in your arms, you'll be happy with the outcome, so it's not even worth the worry.

You can control so many other things during your pregnancy, and you should focus on those. These tasks will help you be productive and keep you from worrying about things beyond your control. In addition to taking care of yourself, things you can control include:

- buying, washing, and putting away baby clothes
- preparing and freezing meals for later
- bonding with your baby

6. BE PATIENT WITH YOURSELF

Remember to be patient with yourself during pregnancy. It can be easy to feel like you should know everything since you're the one carrying the baby, but that's not realistic. True, your body will naturally do what it needs to do to make sure your baby is healthy as it grows, but you're not expected to know everything all at once. Every day is a chance to learn and grow, so give yourself that grace.

You might feel like you need to do everything and learn everything before your baby is born, but you don't want to overload yourself. Remember to take it a day at a time and make manageable tasks for yourself. Maybe you'll read a chapter of this book every day; that's a great way to learn more each day without overwhelming yourself. Perhaps you'll research a specific question each week or try to complete some of your nesting tasks each week. Though you have a timeline with your pregnancy, there's no need to feel like you're racing to the finish line.

Having patience with yourself will set you up for success. Instead of pushing yourself to complete twelve major tasks each day, slowing down and making progress towards a few of the more urgent tasks will help you reach each goal and ensure you're doing good work in the meantime.

Patience is especially crucial during pregnancy because of how your energy will ebb and flow. You can't push yourself to do so many things every day because you might be more exhausted tomorrow than you are today. Being patient will help you adapt to each day as it comes, and it will also help you be self-aware. This level of self-awareness works hand-in-hand with mindfulness because you're accepting your state of being and energy levels as they are, without trying to push yourself to the unattainable.

7. REMEMBER YOUR END GOAL

Being patient also helps you remember your end goal. Instead of racing towards the finish line, you're taking steps to enjoy the entire process. You know you're going to have a baby at the end of this, so why not slow down and enjoy the journey? This is your first pregnancy, and you're about to become a mom; there's some magic bubbling beneath the surface that seems so exciting if you just let yourself feel it.

This pregnancy, in particular, is something you'll never experience again in your life. You're on the cusp of becoming a parent and changing the path of your life, and that's a major goal to look forward to! That's why so much of this mental and emotional health journey focuses on journaling, being mindful, and processing your emotions. Becoming a parent for the first time is like nothing you've experienced in your life up to this point. It can feel surreal to look around you and realize that everything will be different in a few short months.

Thinking about the end goal is different than focusing on the future. There are no worries associated with remembering your end goal. You're not thinking about what type of mother you'll be or how you'll pay for college. Thinking about the goal is all about relishing the feeling of knowing you're going to become a parent and hold your baby in your arms. There is only excitement and curiosity when you think of your goal, not worries about the possible negative outcomes of the situation. This is a positive thinking exercise that builds you up to be excited about finally having your baby in your arms after so many months of preparing.

8. ENJOY BEING INTIMATE WITH YOUR PARTNER

Every pregnant woman is different when it comes to her comfort level of being affectionate during pregnancy. Those feelings often change due to hormones and the stage of pregnancy, as well. But whenever possible, enjoy being intimate with your partner. This is the last period where just the two of you are in the world! While you and your partner might focus much of your time preparing your lives for this change, you should also spend some time connecting on an intimate level.

Of course, while we're talking about hormonal changes, we have to talk about sex! There will be times during pregnancy when you feel so sexy and can't keep your hands off your partner. Make sure to take advantage of these moments. Both of you will feel better after being intimate, and it will strengthen your relationship as well. Plus, it's physical activity, so it can count as some moderate exercise!

Being intimate isn't only about sex. Go on dates whenever possible. Watch some of your favorite movies and shows together to relax. Spend time in bed being together, touching, and talking. Make sure you're spending as much time together as you can. You created a baby together, so now you can use these last few months as a twosome to truly enjoy each other. Your family is growing and will change for the better, but you'll never get back these days of being a couple on the brink of parenthood. You can share so many emotions and experiences in this time to strengthen your intimate bond and relationship.

9. COUNT YOUR BLESSINGS

Pregnancy is a great time to practice gratitude by counting your blessings. Think of everything you have in life to be thankful for. This includes thinking of experiences you've been through that brought you to where you are now.

Counting your blessings can include looking around your house and appreciating all that you have. You might want to do this as an exercise with your partner and take turns saying aloud what you're thankful for. This can include characteristics you possess as well! You might be grateful for a safe place to bring your baby home. You can also share that you're thankful to have a supportive partner that cooks dinner every night.

Even negatives from your past can be reframed as something to be thankful for. Maybe you stopped smoking when you discovered you were pregnant. You can frame that as being grateful for your baby helping you get healthy, even though that addiction can be so hard to kick. Most likely, the attributes that you've developed to become the amazing mother that you will be can be traced back to positive and negative experiences from your past. Everything you've experienced will help you be a better parent for your child, and they can learn from your lessons as well.

Maybe you're grateful that your parents raised you with strong values you can pass along to your child. If your parents are still alive, call or visit them to share this gratitude. They'll love knowing that the choices they made when you were young have impacted you in this way. After all, you're about to be a parent now, too. Every parent worries about damaging their child in some way, so if you have a chance to tell your parents how grateful you are for them, let them know!

10. USE POSITIVE AFFIRMATIONS

Positive affirmations can help you see the positive during your pregnancy. You can use these as mantras you recite when you're practicing yoga or having a mindful moment. They enable you to appreciate all your body is doing to benefit you and your baby. These affirmations also help you stay focused on the good things when your mind might be trying to take you into a spiral of worry.

If you're feeling negative about your changing body, try some of these affirmations:

- My body is a safe vessel for my baby.
- My pregnancy is beautiful.
- My body is nourishing my baby.
- I'm not going to be pregnant forever.
- My body is strong enough to carry my baby.
- I am listening to what my body needs.
- My body is equipped to give birth.

If you're consumed with worry about the future, try these affirmations:

- I have a great purpose on this earth.
- I am here to be the best for my baby.

- I am taking it one day at a time.
- I am making the best decisions for my baby and me.
- My baby feels my love.
- My baby and I are healthy and strong.
- I am doing everything I can to be ready to parent my baby.
- My life will be better because my baby will be a part of it.

If an affirmation doesn't feel right to you, don't push it! The good thing about affirmations is you can find one to suit what you're feeling at the moment. If none of these seem right, focus on the issue that is bothering you. Is it body image? Health? Your capabilities as a mother? Take one of your worries and structure a positive statement around it. Even if you don't believe it at the moment, say it with force, like you're willing it to be true! After all, a positive affirmation is just a way of reminding yourself of the truth. Once you start saying it, you'll start believing it, and then you'll start living it.

11. BE AWARE OF YOUR THOUGHTS

All of this positivity isn't just for you because your thoughts also affect your unborn baby. Even while your baby is growing inside of you, they are a sensitive person who will have a powerful connection with you and the world you're bringing them into. It's been proven that babies who feel optimism and love in the womb are born having fewer mental problems (Nierenberg, 2017).

Neuroscientist and Stanford researcher Bruce Lipton, Ph.D., has found that genes are not set in stone, and they do not determine your child's destiny (Gustafson, 2017). Environmental influences modify genes, and those influences include nutrition, stress, and emotions. These genes, in turn, can be passed on to future generations. So what you think and feel during your pregnancy can influence your baby, your baby's babies, and so on!

Most soon-to-be parents know that their baby can hear them in the womb and notice light patterns, so it's important to talk to your baby and start the phases of daytime and nighttime lighting to encourage natural sleep patterns. But those are external sources, so it makes sense your baby can sense them.

Lipton's research has helped psychologists realize that qualities your baby might exhibit later in life can be traced back to their time in the womb. This includes their confidence levels, propensity for depression, and addictive behaviors. Lipton has even stated in his research that it's true "[t]hat growth-promoting awareness and intention can produce a smarter, healthier and happier baby" (Gustafson, 2017). So it might be easy to wave away positive thinking exercises as fluffy or "woo-woo," but science has proven they work. You might as well set your baby up for success while still in the womb, especially since you will also benefit from this positivity!

Being aware of your thoughts doesn't mean that every thought needs to be a happy one. Negative thoughts are natural, and you especially can't avoid them with so much uncertainty in your life. Instead of preventing yourself from having negative thoughts or punishing yourself for having one, reframe your negative thinking into a positive.

If you think, "I know I won't be a good mother because I'm clearly selfish since I'm struggling to give up my old life," stop and sit with that thought as you reframe it. Instead of seeing that as selfish, acknowledge that it is a hard transition for anyone to go through. Then think, "I've lived for myself for so long that it will take time to adjust to putting my baby first, but I know I can do it." You're restating the negative thought as something neutral: it is hard to change your life after living it a certain way for so long. Then you're adding something powerful and empowering at the end: "I know I can do it." Giving yourself this grace in terms of reality and pushing toward positivity will help you prepare for your baby.

7

PHYSICALLY, EMOTIONALLY, AND MENTALLY PREPARING FOR THE BABY

After spending so much time getting used to your pregnant body and making the most welcoming environment for your baby, both inside and out, it's finally time to prepare for your baby's arrival into the world! There are certain changes you'll go through as you get closer to delivery, including physical, emotional, and mental changes. Here's what to look out for.

PHYSICALLY

Your body will let you know when it's getting closer to time to have your baby. In the movies, it's always a big moment like a woman's water breaking or experiencing painful contractions, but that doesn't always happen in real life. Your body will slowly make changes to prepare itself for smooth childbirth, and you can be on the lookout for these shifts long before you feel the first contraction.

You'll have an idea of when your baby will come based on the due date, but those are usually just estimates based on your last period and how your baby is developing. Your due date can be off by as much as two weeks, but just know that most women give birth between 38 and 42 weeks, with 40 weeks qualifying as a standard, full-term pregnancy.

Many women notice their energy levels change when they're about to give birth. A woman who has been enjoying high-energy days might suddenly feel lethargic even a week in advance. Other women will get a burst of energy and feel like they're able to accomplish everything they need to do before the baby arrives. If you notice a drastic change in your energy a few days to a week in advance of your due date, it might be a sign that your baby is on the way!

Your baby will also drop lower into your pelvis as it prepares to be born. This shift is called lightening because you're able to breathe easier once the baby has moved, so your whole body will feel lighter.

After you feel your baby shift like this, you'll know that both you and the baby are ready to meet!

Some women lose their mucus plug a few days before going into labor. This is the plug that sealed your cervix while the baby grew. When it is discharged, it's a way your body is opening the path for the baby to be born. Not all women see their mucus plug, but if you do, be warned that it might be pink or blood-streaked. It can be alarming to see this on your underpants or when you wipe, but it's normal. If you're worried about how yours looks, always err on the side of caution and contact your doctor for reassurance.

The first contractions you feel will be irregular. They happen as your cervix starts to soften and thin so the baby can come through. Your cervix will begin to dilate slowly at first, but as you and your baby are ready for labor, it will open more quickly, and you'll experience stronger and longer contractions.

When you first start feeling contractions, try to keep track of how long they last and how far apart they are. This will help your doctor know how soon the baby will be born. Contractions can be irregular for a while, and early labor can be unpredictable in terms of how long it lasts. With your first baby, early labor can even last for days as your body prepares to give birth! While you're in early labor, you can do things you normally would, especially if these tasks help you relax. You might want to go for a walk, practice breathing exercises, take a warm bath, or try to distract yourself with a book or movie.

It might feel like early labor is stretching out with no end in sight, but don't stress about its duration. Just monitor your contractions because once they become regular and intense, it'll be time to go to the hospital to have the baby.

Early labor is your body preparing itself to give birth, and active labor is when things really start to happen. Your cervix will be dilating enough for the baby to come out, and you'll most likely be experiencing strong, frequent contractions. You might feel nauseous or vomit from the pain radiating from your back as your body shifts to give birth. You can also feel your legs cramp up, so make sure you're not at risk of falling.

Your water may break when your baby is ready to come into the world, but some women don't have this happen before active labor. Other women might need their doctor or midwife to rupture their amniotic sac for them. But if your water breaks before delivery, you'll most likely be going into labor in the next 24 hours.

Active labor can take anywhere from four to eight hours or longer. Women typically dilate at one centimeter per hour, but if your water breaks or you're experiencing strong contractions, you'll want to go ahead and go to the hospital, so you'll be in your doctor's care.

Since this is your first baby, you might be nervous about how to tell signs of delivery from false labor. Usually, irregular contractions mean you're experiencing false labor. While true contractions can be irregular at first, they start lasting the same duration and increase in frequency with time. False labor contractions are entirely unpredictable and don't increase in length or occurrence. You might also be feeling these contractions at the front of your belly, which could just be related to the baby moving. Contractions that are preparing you for labor are felt from the lower back and in your groin.

If you've gone past your due date, your doctor will have advice on what to do. Don't try any of the old wives' tales about drinking castor oil to help the baby slide out! Sometimes, being active can help, like going on long walks or being intimate with your partner, but your doctor will know best. Sometimes, there's nothing to do but wait.

EMOTIONALLY

You've been on an emotional roller coaster ride throughout your pregnancy, so don't expect it to be any easier when you're giving birth. Everything you've been waiting for is happening, so it's going to feel like a waterfall mix of anxiety and relief.

Breathing is such a big part of labor that you'll already be primed for it from your mindfulness breathing exercises. Since you've been using your breath to calm you down, it'll work double-duty for you as you're giving birth. You'll be able to breathe to focus on pushing and delivering oxygen to your baby, and you'll also be able to use it to calm yourself down. Well, as much as you can be calm during delivery!

Giving birth is so emotional that it's normal to feel fragile at this time. You have so much going on while you're in early and active labor that trying to regulate your emotions shouldn't be a big concern. If you feel like crying, let yourself cry! This is such a significant event in your life that you should give yourself the grace to feel any emotion that washes over you.

If at all possible, try to repair any damaged relationships before you give birth. This is especially important if the relationship is with your partner or a family member, but it also can encompass friends. People will be around a lot to see the baby, and you don't want things to be awkward if you can help it at all. It might seem like a major feat when you're still pregnant and experiencing so many different hormonal changes, but try to look ahead and think of how relieved and peaceful you'll feel after giving birth. That goodwill is a feeling you can imagine now and use to let go of any grudges you're holding against important people in your life. If you're resenting them for things that happened in the past, try to talk about it with them. If nothing else, try to forgive them now so this negativity doesn't surround your birth and your time with your newborn.

That doesn't mean you need to let other people walk all over you. If someone wants to be in the delivery room while you're giving birth and you're not okay with it, don't suck it up to keep the peace. This is a time when you're going to be working hard physically and going through so much emotionally that you want to be surrounded by those you truly care about. If that's just your partner and medical team, so be it. Everyone else can meet the baby later. Your priority during delivery is you, and everyone else needs to accept that.

That being said, you won't be able to control your birth completely. Restricting who can be in the hospital room with you is one thing, but your baby may have other ideas. Your birth plan might not go as you initially hoped, and you need to come to terms with that possibility before you're actually in active labor. Trying to push your baby out while also coping with a major change in your best-laid plans is going to make an emotional wreck out of you. Instead, know that the birth plan you make is what will happen in an ideal world. Other than that, whatever happens to get your baby out safely should be your only concern. And even that shouldn't be your concern because you have your doctor and medical team taking care of that aspect.

You can talk about your birth plan with your doctor early in your pregnancy. Tell the team how you'd like for your birth to go. If you're set on having a natural birth with no drugs, your doctor can give you an idea of how that will feel and what you can do during your pregnancy to help facilitate that type of birth. You can ask for your doctor's input about many aspects of your delivery, but it's important to be realistic. It can be hard to talk about what might happen when you're nowhere near giving birth, but asking early on will give you time to accept the idea. Many women's deliveries don't go according to their birth plans, and your doctor can verify this, so you don't need to feel like a failure if yours doesn't go according to plan.

At the same time, it might help to talk to your doctor about different options. Say you want the natural birth with no drugs. If the pain gets too bad at a point, can you ask for drugs? If the baby isn't coming naturally, what happens then? Sometimes knowing the steps to an alternative birth will soften the blow of not having the birth plan you want. You'll still be aware of what is happening, step by step, even if it's not what you initially wanted. Being informed about the possibilities can be empowering and prevent you from being too distressed during labor.

Sometimes having a different birth from what you expected won't hit you until the trauma has ended. It's okay to mourn the fact that you didn't get the birth you dreamed of but channel those positive thinking tips into this area of your life as well. Look at the baby you're holding in your arms, the ultimate end goal, and be grateful for all you have. Your body performed a miraculous feat to deliver this baby, even if it didn't go according to plan. Appreciate what you have and what you've been through, then look forward to your happy future with your baby.

MENTALLY

Remember, emotions are your gut reactions to things that are happening and how you feel about those reactions. Your mental health while giving birth relies more on feeling ready. No matter how much you've prepared your home life, being ready is just a state of mind. It means you've accepted where you are and the fact that your baby is coming, and you're here for it.

You've already done so much work throughout this book and your entire pregnancy that there is no doubt you're ready to give birth. It can seem intimidating because it's a big unknown. This is your first baby, and all of the movies and medical dramas you've seen can't prepare you for how your delivery experience is actually going to go. That's when you have to trust in yourself. You've educated yourself as much as you can, and there's definitely such a thing as too much information! At a certain point, you can't read any more about how to care for your body during pregnancy or what will happen in each stage of labor. You've got the information you need, and you're ready for it. Now, you're just waiting.

Remember all of this information as you're going into early labor. This is the time when you can feel your body shifting, priming itself to give birth to your baby. Remember that you have learned all you can to feel prepared for what's going to happen. You are strong and capable, and your body is going to do its best to safely usher your baby into this world, just as it's been taking care of your baby for the last nine months.

When you're feeling such extreme pains coursing through your body during active labor, it can be so easy to think (and say!), "I can't do this!" It can all feel like too much. But your mental readiness can over-power your physical pain. Tell yourself that you know you can do it, you trust your body, you've been building your health and strength for nine months, and now, you're going to see it all pay off during childbirth.

While your mental state will significantly differ from when you're pregnant to when you're giving birth, you're still the same person at your core. You're just as strong during labor as you were when you felt empowered and prepared a week ago. You still have everything set up at home and ready for the baby. There's no reason to doubt what you already know. While the uncertainty of giving birth can feel overwhelming, trust in yourself.

Mindfulness can come in handy in terms of keeping your mental state calm during labor. If you meditate, practice mindfulness, or think of positive affirmations during labor, your baby will come into the world feeling safe and protected by your positivity. Being positive also increases your endorphin levels, which will help relieve pain during labor.

The positive affirmations shared in the last chapter can help your mental well-being during early and active labor. You can even share some of the more empowering affirmations with your partner and birth team so they can help psych you back up if you're feeling drained and overwhelmed.

8

STAYING PHYSICALLY, EMOTIONALLY, AND MENTALLY HEALTHY DURING THE FIRST MONTHS OF POSTPARTUM

Giving birth can feel like an immense relief. Everything you've been working toward for the past nine months has finally happened. You have your sweet newborn in your arms. You get to bring your baby home and introduce them to your loved ones. You change your daily routine to center around the feeding and caring of your baby. It can be a magical time as you bond with your baby, but even the most prepared new parents feel like they exist in a haze.

New mothers have an especially tough time adapting to these changes after giving birth. You often think that pregnancy ends after you have the baby, and your life goes back to normal with a baby added to the mix. But in recent years, medical professionals have added a fourth trimester onto the pregnancy experience. This means that you'll experience physical, emotional, and mental changes during the first three months postpartum, just like you did during the previous three trimesters and when giving birth.

PHYSICAL

After you have your baby, there are undoubtedly many physical aspects you have to adapt to and heal from before you can get anything resembling your old body back. Your uterus will contract back to its previous size, which might cause you to experience some mild contractions or cramps. Your belly will start to go back to its original size as well.

Even after giving birth, you might experience some swelling in your face, feet, and hands as you did during pregnancy. Make sure you're drinking plenty of water, wear loose clothes, and try to put your feet up as much as possible. Sleeping on your left side instead of your back can also help the swelling go down naturally.

After giving birth vaginally, you might have a dark discharge called lochia. This is your body eliminating the extra blood inside the uterus for your baby and isn't cause for alarm. The lochia will ebb and flow throughout the day, with more being present when you get up in the morning, when you're physically active, and when you're breastfeeding. If you had a cesarean section (C-section), you might have less lochia just 24 hours after delivery.

For the first three days, lochia will be dark red and thick. After the fourth day, the discharge will start to lighten in color, and by the end of two weeks, it will be yellowish and thin. It should stop completely anywhere from four to six weeks after giving birth. Wear pads to catch the discharge, not tampons—nothing should be inserted into your vagina for six weeks after labor to allow for healing.

If you gave birth naturally, you might have had an episiotomy, where the doctor surgically cut your vagina to prevent tearing during labor. This cut can heal on its own, or you might have stitches. Either way, care for your perineal area carefully because it's a wound that can be painful and sensitive. You can take a warm sitz bath to relieve the discomfort.

You'll be given a peri bottle to keep the area clean after using the bathroom. Fill this bottle with warm water, then spray it on your perineal area every time you use the toilet. Pat the area dry with toilet paper, but don't rub it. Apply a clean pad to your underwear each time you go to the bathroom. You'll have to keep this up for about a week after giving birth.

If you're experiencing perineum soreness even when the area is clean, consider wrapping an ice pack in a towel and applying it to the area. You can also soak a cotton pad in witch hazel and freeze it for additional comfort and cleanliness. You might want to sit on a pillow or donut-shaped cushion for extra softness and support instead of sitting directly on hard furniture. The tips for perineal pain can also apply to hemorrhoids, which you might continue experiencing after having your baby.

If you had a C-section, you might have drainage from the incision. You'll have to treat this wound as you would a major surgery, even though you'll still have to care for your newborn. It's important to rest as much as possible to allow this incision to heal. You can wash it with soap and warm water to keep it clean and remove the drainage.

Whether you're breastfeeding or not, your breasts will become engorged, and it can be painful. It might make your breasts feel hard to heavy. If you're breastfeeding, this discomfort might mean it's time to feed your baby. If the baby isn't hungry, you can pump milk to relieve the pain. If you're not breast-feeding, you can ask your doctor for pain medication to ease the engorgement. Ice packs might also help numb the pain.

No matter what, make sure you're wearing a supportive bra, so you don't experience additional discomfort. You can also take warm showers to help the milk let down and then feed your baby immediately.

If you're leaking milk or other discharge, you can wear breast pads to keep your bra dry and prevent stains on your clothing. Even if you're not able to breastfeed your baby, you might experience some leaking from your breasts for a week or two after giving birth.

If you're concerned about any leaking or breast pain, consult your doctor. It's possible to get infections in your milk ducts, so you'll want to ensure your baby is getting all of the milk they need without putting your health at risk.

After giving birth naturally, you might experience some changes when it comes to urinating and having bowel movements. You can feel squeamish at the thought of wiping or pushing too hard for a bowel movement, but a normal level of exertion is okay and shouldn't cause you additional pain. If you continue eating a healthy diet with fruits and vegetables and drink plenty of water, your bowel movements should stay regular. If you're worried about pushing too hard, ask your doctor for a stool softener so you won't be uncomfortable.

For a few days after birth, you might feel some discomfort when urinating, but that should involve no pain or burning. If that's what you're experiencing, contact your doctor.

You might experience incontinence after giving birth since your muscles have stretched. You can continue the Kegel exercises taught in chapter three to strengthen these muscles. Any incontinence you experience should improve a few weeks after giving birth.

As your hormones level out, you might find yourself sweating more than usual, even more so at night. Make sure you drink plenty of water during this time to keep yourself hydrated, especially if you're breastfeeding. Shower regularly so all of your healing wounds can stay clean and change your bed sheets frequently, so they're clean and will help you get a good night's sleep.

If you're bottle-feeding your baby, you might get your first period as soon as six weeks after giving birth. If you're breastfeeding, you may not get a period until your baby is weaned, though you can still get pregnant during this time. Whether you're bottle-feeding or breastfeeding, your first few periods after having a baby might be irregular, but that is nothing to worry about.

EMOTIONAL

Your emotions have been up and down for the past nine months, but you're not likely to get much stability from them soon. Giving birth is an amazing experience, and you're likely to feel happy and delighted holding your newborn in your arms, anxious about being a parent once you leave the hospital, and maybe even depressed because of your hormonal crash.

You might feel like you need to put your life on hold as you adjust to being a new mother. While it's not as extreme as that, it's not a bad idea to limit the tasks you take on that don't revolve around caring for your baby and allowing your body to heal. Even having visitors over to see the baby can be emotionally taxing, so it's okay to limit visitors to one a day or have a set time limit for their stay.

As many as eight out of 10 new mothers report feeling depressed after giving birth, so don't beat yourself up if you're one of the eight. With your hormones trying to level out while you stress over caring for your newborn, these negative thoughts are bound to happen. You'll probably feel blissfully happy for a couple of days, riding your adrenaline high of giving birth. You might think you've made it through the hormone rampage, but the baby blues typically don't hit until the third or fourth day. It's as if your emotions are trying to lull you into a false sense of security before dragging you down into the negativity.

If you're only experiencing baby blues, they should dissipate within two weeks. That doesn't make these emotions any easier to handle at the moment, but knowing they have a time limit can help you see the light at the end of the tunnel. The baby blues might make you feel very impatient and irritable, which you can take out on people around you, especially your partner. You might always feel anxious or on the verge of tears, but you won't feel this way all of the time. These feelings come and go throughout the day. Ensuring you're eating small meals and snacks throughout the day and resting whenever you feel tired can help alleviate the baby blues.

If your baby blues persist beyond two weeks, you might have postpartum depression. Even if you didn't feel the baby blues, you might feel this depression by the fourth week postpartum. Some women have said that their postpartum depression ended when their period returned or when they weaned their baby from breastfeeding.

Postpartum depression can feel like different things to different women. You might feel nervous and anxious, to the point where you can cause yourself to panic. You might feel exhausted all of the time, even if you're not overexerting your body. You might feel more traditional symptoms of depression like sadness and a sense of hopelessness. You might have trouble eating or sleeping and be preoccupied with concern for your baby's well-being. You might feel guilty, inadequate as a mother, or worthless in the scheme of things. Any high or low you feel might be incredibly exaggerated, to the extreme where that's the only emotion you can feel at the time.

These symptoms can appear alone or together and be mild or all-consuming. You can have good days and bad days. Resting whenever you're tired might help. Remember a lot of the positivity tips you depended on during pregnancy; they can still be effective after you've given birth. Focus only on what you can control, and don't push yourself to do everything or to do it perfectly. Stay active and go on walks with your baby. Find other mothers in support groups or at Mommy and Me classes. Try to take it easy in other areas of your life, so you don't have too many significant life changes all happening in a short period.

You don't have to get past these emotions on your own. Talk to your partner and your support system. Seek help if you think it would be beneficial. You can find a therapist to talk to or a psychiatrist to prescribe you helpful medications.

If you ever feel like hurting yourself or your baby, get professional help immediately. You might feel like you're at your worst, but there is help for you. Never think that you're overreacting or taking something too seriously. While baby blues sounds like a cutesy name, those feelings are real, and postpartum depression is an entirely different struggle. One in seven women experience postpartum depression, but even then, it's not widely talked about and still has a negative stigma surrounding it.

Don't even worry about that stigma if you think you're experiencing postpartum depression. Many mothers think this depression is a weakness or a sign that they're not cut out for motherhood, but it's not that at all. It can just be a complication from giving birth, especially when you consider all of the hormones involved in the process. The combination of your body's physical changes with the hormones that go along with them is enough on its own. Still, then you're having emotional issues after the joy of giving birth, the anxiety of becoming a parent, and the sleep deprivation that occurs when you have a newborn.

If you've struggled with depression before pregnancy, make sure your doctor is aware. If you've been on medication before, your doctor might recommend you keep taking it through pregnancy in hopes of preventing postpartum depression. Even if you'd prefer to stop taking meds for your baby's sake, inform your doctor, so you'll have a support system keeping an eye on your symptoms.

If you haven't experienced depression before, you're still at risk for postpartum depression, so you'll want to keep an eye on any potential symptoms. Even if you're experiencing mild symptoms, you'll want to tell your doctor and possibly get professional help. If you feel depressed, don't be embarrassed to talk about it with someone. Know that everyone is rooting for you because you've just been through an incredible pregnancy journey and given birth to a beautiful baby. No one wants to shame you for what you might be going through, so seek help. If you're feeling depressed for longer than two weeks and don't feel like you're getting better, you'll want to seek help.

MENTAL

Remember, emotions are the way you're reacting to things that come your way. Your mental health can be influenced by how you process these emotions. It can be hard to separate yourself from your emotions when you're a new mother juggling so many other things, but taking some time to be diplomatic about what you're going through can help.

First of all, realize that everything you're going through is normal. What you see new mothers going through on TV shows and in movies is greatly exaggerated. Even the mothers you see in your own community might seem like they have it all together, but everyone feels like they're grasping at straws at this point. Even if they do make it look effortless, it isn't worth comparing yourself to them.

You also don't need to feel that bond with your baby instantly. Many women do because they've spent nine months carrying the baby around, so they feel used to having a constant companion.

There is a big difference between carrying a newborn in your stomach and having a live baby that you need to care for constantly. It's understandable if it takes you time to feel something for that little person. After all, you just met!

Unfortunately, society makes it seem like all mothers will instantly love their baby and know how to care for it. If you have those natural mothering instincts, enjoy them! They can be a great help and can make you feel confident as a new parent, but that doesn't mean not feeling that immediate love for your baby makes you a monster. Society, your friends, and even your family might make it seem that way, but there is no shame in needing time to adjust to your baby. You will have plenty of time to bond with your child and fall in love with them.

Mourning your old life goes beyond being an emotion at this stage because you're already deep into a new lifestyle. Even if you have time to step away and process your life with your baby, and even if you love that life, it's okay to miss what you had before. Talk to parents of older children and teenagers, and they'll tell you the same! You can love your child and be excited to raise them, but you can mourn your old life at the same time. It doesn't mean you want to go back to it; you can just admit it was good and is hard to get over.

This mourning can include missing how your relationship was when it was only you and your partner. It might have been much easier to live with just the two of you. Constantly caring for the baby might take its toll on the relationship you have with your partner. You might have more arguments than before because you're still trying to balance your postpartum emotions, and as the mother, you might feel like you know best when it comes to the baby. But for your mental health (and that of your partner and others around you), it can help to step back and let other people pick up the slack.

It can also help your mental well-being to realize that you can't do everything on your own, and others are willing to step up and help. Having the baby does not mean that you will instantly feel 100% prepared! Remember, all you can do is focus on what you can control. You never know what's around the corner as you're raising a child, so you can be prepared to the best of your abilities, and otherwise, be flexible. You're along for the ride at this point, so it's healthier for your mind if you relinquish some degree of control and accept what's coming.

CONCLUSION

Congratulations on progressing through this journey! This book gave you a lot of practical information, but the last section was especially heavy, so it's important to remember that you can do this! You are capable and strong, and you have taken control of the situation by reading this guide and empowering yourself even further.

From changing your diet and starting exercise early in your pregnancy, you've strengthened your body to not only be healthy for you and your baby but also to prepare it for childbirth. In the chapters about labor and postpartum, you can see how important it is to eat right and do exercises—especially Kegels!

Improving your health will also boost your mental and emotional well-being, so it's nice to know that every positive change you make during pregnancy will benefit you and your baby. Getting in tune with your body while you're pregnant will ensure you're able to listen to what it needs even after you give birth.

If you're having doubts about your ability to be a mother, know that you're not alone. No woman has it all together at this stage of her pregnancy, but you're doing great work to figure it out ahead of time with this guide. Arming yourself with this knowledge is a great foundation, and remember, your doctor is always available to help you with any questions or concerns you may have along the way.

I think the biggest thing to remember as you go from being an expectant parent to a new mother is that you can do this! You are capable and curious, so you'll always be willing to learn and make the best choices for your baby. Taking steps to understand more about your body, health, and growing baby during pregnancy shows how much you already care for your little one.

It's also important to be realistic in your expectations for your pregnancy and parenthood. Society will make you think something is natural and expected, but it doesn't have to be that way. One of the worst things you can do during pregnancy is compare yourself to others. Your body knows what it's doing, and you will adjust to these changes naturally. Don't worry about what other mothers are doing in their lives or thinking about your life—trust yourself!

While this book is geared toward first-time moms, there's a lot of information you can come back to if you have another child in the future. The knowledge is meant to soothe new mothers because there is so much unknown about having your first child, but each pregnancy is so different that it's worth revisiting this guide if you need to. You might find that some tips and tricks help you with certain aspects of future pregnancy in different ways than they did when you were expecting your first. There is comfort in knowing that you have a guide to help you through your pregnancies.

So much of the advice is practical to apply to your everyday life as well. The exercises might be geared towards pregnant women, but studies have shown that Kegels can help women throughout their lives, even beyond menopause! And healthy eating is always a great choice. If you want to eat a balanced diet without following a fad diet, the selections from the five food groups can help you make good choices.

I hope the positive thinking sections are some that you'll take away. I think they're crucial because they can help so much during pregnancy as your hormones fluctuate, but they can also help you a lot on your parenting journey. Keeping a level head as you deal with a child has so much value. If you can balance that with mindfulness and time for yourself, you'll find that parenthood can be more calm and productive than you ever thought possible!

If this book helped you during your pregnancy journey, prepare for labor, and make it through the fourth trimester, please leave a review on Amazon so that other expectant mothers can benefit from the knowledge. If any piece of advice, in particular, helped you through, I'd love to hear about it! Sharing our knowledge is an excellent way of building a supportive community of mothers, so please consider leaving reviews for others to benefit from.

AFTERWORD

I WOULD BE INCREDIBLY THANKFUL IF YOU COULD TAKE 60 SECONDS AND LEAVE A BRIEF REVIEW ON AMAZON!